Promoting Psychological Resilience in the U.S. Military

LISA S. MEREDITH • CATHY D. SHERBOURNE

SARAH GAILLOT • LYDIA HANSELL • HANS V. RITSCHARD

ANDREW M. PARKER • GLENDA WRENN

Prepared for the Office of the Secretary of Defense

Approved for public release; distribution unlimited

Center for Military Health Policy Research

A JOINT ENDEAVOR OF RAND HEALTH AND THE
RAND NATIONAL DEFENSE RESEARCH INSTITUTE

The research reported here was sponsored by the Office of the Secretary of Defense (OSD). The research was conducted jointly by the Center for Military Health Policy Research, a RAND Health program, and the Forces and Resources Policy Center, a RAND National Defense Research Institute (NDRI) program. NDRI is a federally funded research and development center sponsored by OSD, the Joint Staff, the Unified Combatant Commands, the Navy, the Marine Corps, the defense agencies, and the defense Intelligence Community under Contract W74V8H-06-C-0002.

Library of Congress Control Number: 2011931851

ISBN: 978-0-8330-5063-2

Cover design by Eileen Delson La Russo
Cover photo by Tech. Sgt. Cecilio M. Ricardo Jr. (U.S. Air Force)

Published 2011 by the RAND Corporation
1776 Main Street, P.O. Box 2138, Santa Monica, CA 90407-2138
1200 South Hayes Street, Arlington, VA 22202-5050
4570 Fifth Avenue, Suite 600, Pittsburgh, PA 15213-2665
RAND URL: http://www.rand.org/
To order RAND documents or to obtain additional information, contact
Distribution Services: Telephone: (310) 451-7002;
Fax: (310) 451-6915; Email: order@rand.org

Preface

The operational tempo associated with the conflicts in Iraq and Afghanistan creates a number of challenges for service members and their families. Service members have been deploying for extended periods on a repeated basis, which, combined with the other consequences of combat, may challenge their and their families' ability to cope with the stress of deployment. While most military personnel and their families cope well under these difficult circumstances, many will also experience difficulties handling stress at some point.

There are, however, a growing number of programs and strategies provided by the military and civilian sectors to encourage and support psychological resilience to stress for service members and families. Psychological resilience is defined as the capacity to adapt successfully in the presence of risk and adversity. Previous research from the field of psychology delineating the factors that foster psychological resilience is available, but we do not know whether and how well the current military resilience programs are addressing these factors in their activities. Further, there is little known about the effectiveness of these programs on developing resilience.

To assist the Department of Defense (DoD) in understanding methodologies that could be useful in promoting resilience among service members and their families, the RAND National Defense Research Institute (RAND NDRI) conducted a focused literature review to identify factors that were supported by the literature (e.g., evidence-informed) for promoting psychological resilience. The study also included a review of a subset of resilience programs to determine the extent to which they included those evidence-informed factors. This monograph describes the context, approach, and findings from these research activities. It will be of interest to researchers and policymakers in the military community concerned with programming to promote health and prevent negative consequences of war on the nation's service members and their families.

This research was sponsored by the Office of the Assistant Secretary of Defense for Health Affairs (OASD/HA) and conducted jointly by RAND Health's Center for Military Health Policy Research and the Forces and Resources Policy Center of the RAND National Defense Research Institute (NDRI). The Center for Military Health Policy Research taps RAND expertise in both defense and health policy to conduct research for the Department of Defense, the Veterans Administration, and nonprofit organizations. RAND Health aims to transform the well-being of all people by solving complex problems in health and health care. NDRI is a federally funded research and development center sponsored by the Office of the Secretary of Defense, the Joint Staff, the Unified Combatant Commands, the Navy, the Marine Corps, the defense agencies, and the defense Intelligence Community.

For more information on the Center for Military Health Policy Research, see http://www.rand.org/multi/military/ or contact the co-directors (contact information is provided on the web page). For more information on the Forces and Resources Policy Center, see http://www.rand.org/nsrd/about/frp.html or contact the director (contact information is provided on the web page).

Contents

Figures

Tables

Summary

Study Background, Purpose, and Approach

The long and frequent deployments of U.S. armed forces associated with Operation Iraqi Freedom (OIF) and Operation Enduring Freedom (OEF), combined with the other consequences of combat, such as exposure to trauma, have tested the resilience and coping skills of U.S. military service members and their families. While most military personnel and families are resilient under these difficult circumstances, many also experience difficulties handling stress at some point.

Psychological resilience refers to the process of coping with or overcoming exposure to adversity or stress. With regard to mental health interventions, psychological resilience is more than an individual personality trait—it is a process involving interaction among an individual, that individual's life experiences, and current life context. For example, resilience can apply to contexts relevant either to prevention (before exposure to stress) or to treatment (when recovering from the harmful effects of such stress).

Over the past several years, DoD has implemented a number of programs and strategies to promote psychological resilience among service members. Although the value of resilience programming is widely accepted, little is known empirically about the programs' effectiveness or the extent to which they are based on factors identified by social and behavioral science as contributing to resilience in individuals or groups. Although some previous research has shed light on the factors that foster psychological resilience, this research has typically not been assembled in a summary form that can be used easily to design programs. Moreover, previous research has not fully examined how these factors might apply in the military.

To assist DoD in understanding factors and methodologies that are informed by social and psychological research and may be useful in promoting psychological resilience in service members and their families, RAND NDRI conducted a study to identify evidence-informed practices for promoting factors that foster psychological resilience. The study also assessed selected resilience programs to determine whether they incorporate evidence-informed practices to promote resilience and includes a literature review and a program review.

Factors That Promote Resilience: Findings from the Literature Review

Using the working definition of psychological resilience specified above, we conducted a systematic review of the scientific literature on psychological resilience. The review had a twofold purpose:

- to identify evidence-informed factors that promote psychological resilience (i.e., resilience factors)
- to assess the strength of the evidence base associated with each factor.

We identified 270 relevant publications. The initial set of evidence-informed factors for promoting psychological resilience, based on these publications, was identified by the research team. These evidence-informed factors were confirmed by an expert review process, yielding 20 evidence-informed factors associated with resilience. We categorized these resilience factors according to whether they operated at the individual, family, organization (or unit), and community levels. We used such an organizing framework to distinguish intrinsic factors that promote resilience within an individual from resilience factors that involve other individuals who are part of a group (e.g., family, organization, community). Each factor is listed and defined below.

Individual-Level Factors
- **Positive coping.** The process of managing taxing circumstances, expending effort to solve personal and interpersonal problems, and seeking to reduce or tolerate stress or conflict, including active/pragmatic, problem-focused, and spiritual[1] approaches to coping
- **Positive affect.** Feeling enthusiastic, active, and alert, including having positive emotions, optimism, a sense of humor (ability to have humor under stress or when challenged), hope, and flexibility about change
- **Positive thinking.** Information processing, applying knowledge, and changing preferences through restructuring, positive reframing, making sense out of a situation, flexibility, reappraisal, refocusing, having positive outcome expectations, a positive outlook, and psychological preparation
- **Realism.** Realistic mastery of the possible, having realistic outcome expectations, self-esteem and self-worth, confidence, self-efficacy, perceived control, and acceptance of what is beyond control or cannot be changed
- **Behavioral control.** The process of monitoring, evaluating, and modifying emotional reactions to accomplish a goal (i.e., self-regulation, self-management, self-enhancement)

---

[1]   Spiritual coping may include the adoption of faith-based beliefs and values as a form of positive coping, receiving support that draws upon those beliefs and values, and also as a form of belongingness through participation in spiritual/faith-based organizations, protocols, ceremonies, etc.

- **Physical fitness.** Bodily ability to function efficiently and effectively in life domains
- **Altruism.** Selfless concern for the welfare of others, motivation to help without reward

Family-Level Factors

- **Emotional ties.** Emotional bonding among family members, including shared recreation and leisure time
- **Communication.** The exchange of thoughts, opinions, or information, including problem-solving and relationship management
- **Support.** Perceiving that comfort is available from (and can be provided to) others, including emotional, tangible, instrumental, informational, and spiritual support
- **Closeness.** Love, intimacy, attachment
- **Nurturing.** Parenting skills
- **Adaptability.** Ease of adapting to changes associated with military life, including flexible roles within the family

Unit-Level Factors

- **Positive command climate.** Facilitating and fostering intra-unit interaction, building pride/support for the mission, leadership, positive role modeling, implementing institutional policies
- **Teamwork.** Work coordination among team members, including flexibility
- **Cohesion.** Unit ability to perform combined actions; bonding together of members to sustain commitment to each other and the mission

Community-Level Factors

- **Belongingness.** Integration, friendships, including participation in spiritual/faith-based organizations, protocols, ceremonies, social services, schools, and so on, and implementing institutional policies
- **Cohesion.** The bonds that bring people together in the community, including shared values and interpersonal belonging
- **Connectedness.** The quality and number of connections with other people in the community; includes connections with a place or people of that place; aspects include commitment, structure, roles, responsibility, and communication
- **Collective efficacy.** Group members' perceptions of the ability of the group to work together

Of the 270 documents that we reviewed:

- There was generally very little rigorous research available across the different resilience factors.
- Only 11 reported results from a randomized design—the strongest form of scientific evidence for intervention effectiveness.
- The individual-level factors with the strongest evidence in the literature were positive thinking, positive affect, positive coping, realism, and behavioral control. These factors were rated as having either moderate evidence (based on cross-sectional correlational or observational design) or strong evidence (based on a randomized design or other longitudinal design).
- Among the family-level factors, family support had the most evidence.
- For unit-level factors, positive command climate had the most evidence.
- For community-level resilience factors, belongingness had the most evidence.

Incorporation of Evidence-Informed Factors in Resilience-Promotion Programs: Findings from Program Review

Next, we examined the extent to which these evidence-informed factors were reflected in resilience-promotion programs relevant to DoD. We conducted interviews with representatives from 23 relevant programs and gathered information about their structure, barriers to implementation and operation that they face, and how the programs assess their effectiveness. Most of the programs were targeted to military members or their families. Every program addressed at least one phase of deployment. Most of the programs delivered these services via workshops or classes, though other forms of services were also provided.

Consistent with the literature review, we found that most programs commonly emphasize one or more of these five individual-level factors: positive thinking, positive coping, behavioral control, positive affect, and realism training. A majority of programs also incorporate positive command climate and teamwork (with less at the unit level). Enhancing family communication was also a relatively widely employed approach to promoting resilience among the programs, though there was less evidence for that family factor than for support. Belongingness was the community factor most widely used by programs.

The most widely cited barriers to program implementation and operations were not specific to resilience factor content and reflect general barriers to implementing novel programs in the military setting. Common barriers include lack of support or "buy-in" from military leadership, logistical issues (such as maintaining adequate staffing, coordinating events, and finding appropriate working space), and lack of sustainable funding. Less commonly reported were barriers specific to implementing resilience content, which were attributed to mental health stigma or difficulty tailoring program content to nonclinical military audiences. Additionally, there are potential barriers to teaching cognitive skills during predeployment because service members are already undergoing rigorous training over very long days and are cognitively depleted because of anxiety and depression associated with anticipating separation and being in harm's way. These conditions make it difficult to find time to practice new skills daily, as recommended. Even among those programs that cited barriers specific to implementing resilience content (such as maintaining interest in stress-related topics, or optimally timing trainings), strong support from leadership was consistently cited as integral to addressing these barriers.

With respect to measuring effectiveness, programs showed considerable variation in their definitions of resilience and the measures they used to gauge program effectiveness. At the individual level, commonly used measures were mental health–related, implying that resilience is defined in terms of the absence of mental health symptoms or conditions such as PTSD, depression, anxiety, and anger. However, others included measures of well-being, positive affect, self-regulation, and mindfulness, reflecting a focus on strengths, rather than deficits. Others focused on performance and functioning, either in general (e.g., using a global assessment tool) or for targeted populations (e.g., reduced productivity for workers, return to duty or reduced training failures for service members). At the family, unit, and community levels, a variety of other measures were used to assess effectiveness of the programs that targeted those populations, including family satisfaction, family communication patterns, unit engagement, and perceived organizational support. No standard measures of resilience or outcomes were used across resilience programs.

We found that only five of the 23 programs had conducted formal assessments of their effectiveness. Because of this, there is limited evidence available as to how well the programs are working or would work if they were implemented in the military. Where evidence is available, the effects appear to be positive but modest. We found that many programs gathered feedback in order to refine and improve their programs. Others have based their programs on years of documented scientific evidence from other studies, which guided the programs' development.

Recommendations for Policy and Programs

Define Resilience

Our literature review identified a variety of resilience definitions, making a summary of the field difficult. Senior commanders and policymakers should carefully formulate a definition of resilience that reflects both the literature and the military culture as a necessary first step in building any existing programs. A clear definition will clarify program stakeholders' understanding of their mission and will also provide clear guidance for those developing program outcome measures.

Integrate Resilience Programming into Policy and Doctrine

For effective implementation of resilience programs, the DoD should consider clear policy to define resilience, to assign roles and responsibilities across the Services, and to provide guidance on program implementation. Because building resilience is largely a function of focused training, such policy could identify the Under Secretary of Defense for Personnel and Readiness as the primary oversight organization for training, implementation, and monitoring. This is important because most resilience researchers are behavioral scientists, whose work would normally inform the military health system; placing responsibility for resilience programs in Health Affairs, however, could possibly hamper implementation of resilience initiatives by operational commanders. Good policy would clearly identify the main factors in building resilience, would properly align oversight with personnel programs, and would allow for flexible implementation that reflects the unique culture of each of the Services.

Strengthen Existing Programs

Evaluation will help to identify strengths and weaknesses of existing programs, possibly aligning with the resilience factors identified here, allowing for improvements to be implemented in an evidence-informed fashion. In addition, randomized controlled trials (RCTs) that compare promising programs with the strongest evidence as well as the current effort to combine programs with the most potential based on current evidence (such as evaluations of the Army's Comprehensive Soldier Fitness (CSF) program, currently underway) are recommended. Finally, additional funding targeted at evaluating existing programs will be needed to accomplish these goals.

Standardize Resilience Measures to Enable Program Comparison

Standardized resilience measures could be applied to a variety of populations in different contexts and allow for a comparison across programs. Such measures would incorporate the evidence-informed factors and could build on or adapt existing metrics of program effectiveness to achieve consensus about what factors comprise resilience, which measures are most valid and reliable for assessing resilience, and their relevance for military populations. This would entail reviewing resilience measures and developing a new resilience measure, based on the overall conceptual structure and list of factors, that is reliable and valid for military populations and their families. The Global Assessment Tool being developed as part of the CSF program for the Army is a step in this direction, although no data on reliability or validity is currently available.

Provide Military Members and Their Families Guidance About the Different Resilience Programs Available

With such a wide variety and rapid increase in programs that are available, it is difficult for individuals to decipher the trade-offs of using different services or programs. A resource guide for resilience programs that compares and contrasts the different types of services offered by different programs would increase awareness about different options.

Incorporate Evidence-Based Resilience Factors

New programs designed to promote resilience should incorporate factors with the most evidence. Thus, the military community will benefit most from programs that teach individual military members and their family members techniques that enhance positive affect, positive thinking, positive coping, realism, and behavioral control. Family-level programs that bolster support, communication, and nurturing; unit-level programs that foster a positive command climate by training military leaders to build mastery and confidence among their troops; and efforts to engage the military community by providing opportunities to participate in integrated activities will likely promote resilience.

Engage Senior Military Leaders

A major challenge to building a resilience program within the military culture is getting support from senior operational leadership. Placing oversight of resilience programs in personnel training programs and training operational commanders to fully understand their role in building a resilience force will help promote values important to the Service cultures. Examples of existing programs include Service career schools for leaders such as the Marine Corps University and the Army's Command and Staff College.

Adopt a Flexible Curriculum

Resilience programs must be designed to dovetail with existing training and community-based programs. At the individual and unit levels, regularly scheduled training should include materials that capture the factors described in this monograph. An excellent example of this is the Marine OSCAR program, which delivers resilience concepts in a format already familiar to Marines alongside existing operational training. Chapel and family programs are ideal examples that promote family and community resilience using existing structures and programs in the community.

Conduct More Rigorous Program Evaluation

Studies with evaluative data need to be encouraged to publish their results. Results from both the literature review and the program review point to the need for more program evaluation. As noted, only 11 documents in the literature review are based on

RCT evaluation design, and only five of the programs reviewed have formally evaluated program success. In general, studies of resilience in the military should enhance scientific rigor by conducting more RCTs and longitudinal studies that span the phases of deployment. This is particularly true for military families, because little research has been published in this area.

Acknowledgments

The authors wish to thank a number of individuals who contributed to this monograph. Four individuals at the DoD's Defense Centers of Excellence for Psychological Health and Traumatic Brain Injury provided helpful guidance and support to the study: LTC Mary Hull, CDR Jerry O'Toole, Mark Bates, and MAJ Todd Yosick. We also thank the expert panelists who vetted the results from the literature review (COL Paul Bartone, Richard Klomp, Hamilton McCubbin, Donald Meichenbaum, CAPT Dori B. Reissman, Steven Southwick, and Froma Walsh) and each of the individuals who we interviewed for our program review. From RAND, we thank Stephanie Taylor for her contribution to the literature review, Terri Tanielian for serving as a project advisor, Dolly Dahdal for help with preparing this monograph, and Nicole Schmidt for help with finalizing some of the program information. We are grateful for David Adamson's thoughtful feedback and suggestions to improve an earlier version of this monograph. We also thank Nora Spiering for her skillful editing, Steve Kistler for publishing guidance, and Matthew Byrd for production editing. Finally, we wish to thank the three peer reviewers, Anita Chandra, Dana Schultz, and John Winkler. Their constructive critiques were addressed, as part of RAND's rigorous quality assurance process, to improve the quality of this monograph.

Abbreviations

ACEP	Army Center for Enhanced Performance
AMEDDC&S	U.S. Army Medical Department Center and School
BH	Behavioral Health
BMI	body mass index
CAPS	Clinician-Administered PTSD Scale
CD-RISC	Connor-Davidson Resilience Scale
CF	Canadian Forces
COSC	(U.S. Marine Corps) Combat Operational Stress Control
CSF	Comprehensive Soldier Fitness
DA	Department of the Army
DCoE	Defense Centers of Excellence for Psychological Health and Traumatic Brain Injury
DoD	Department of Defense
DTIC	Defense Technical Information Center
EEG	electroencephalography
FORSCOM	Forces Command
GAT	Global Assessment Tool
HPI	Human Performance Institute
IRB	institutional review board
IRT	Item Response Theory
JSB	Joint Speakers Bureau

MEDCOM	Medical Command
MMFT	Mindfulness-based Mind Fitness Training
MRS	Marine Resilience Study
MRT	Master Resilience Training
NCO	noncommissioned officer
NDRI	National Defense Research Institute
NSA	National Security Agency
OASD/HA	Office of the Assistant Secretary of Defense for Health Affairs
OEA	Organizational Energy Audit
OEF	Operation Enduring Freedom
OIF	Operation Iraqi Freedom
OSCAR	(U.S. Marine Corps) Operational Stress Control and Readiness
OSI	operational stress injury
OSISS	Operational Stress Injury Social Support
PATHS	Promoting Alternative THinking Strategies
PDHRA	Post-Deployment Health Reassessment Program
POQA	Personal and Organizational Quality Assessment Tool
PPHDP	Preventive Psychological Health Demonstration Project
PRP	The Penn Resiliency Project
PTSD	posttraumatic stress disorder
RAND NDRI	RAND National Defense Research Institute
RCT	randomized controlled trial
REBT	rational emotive behavior therapy
SELF	Soldier Evaluation for Life Fitness
SLWES	Senior Leader Wellness Enhancement Seminar
SMHT	School Mental Health Team
STI-Net	Private Scientific and Technical Network

SWAP	Solider Wellness Assessment Program
SWTP	Spiritual Warrior Training Program
TBI	traumatic brain injury
TRADOC	Training and Doctrine Command
UCSF	University of California, San Francisco
UNC	University of North Carolina
USASOC	U.S. Army Special Operations Command
USD	Under Secretary of Defense
VA	U.S. Department of Veterans Affairs
WBI	Well-Being Index
WRAIR	Walter Reed Army Institute of Research
WRP	Warrior Resiliency Program
WRT	Warrior Resilience and Thriving

CHAPTER ONE

Introduction, Study Objectives, and Approach

Overview and Study Purpose

There has been increasing media attention on the mental health conditions and cognitive impairments that affect many service members participating in Operation Enduring Freedom (OEF) and Operation Iraqi Freedom (OIF). Most military personnel do not return from deployments with these "invisible wounds" (Tanielian and Jaycox, 2008). However, only about half of those who do return with symptoms consistent with a diagnosis of posttraumatic stress disorder (PTSD) or depression see a health care professional for help. In response, former President George W. Bush, Congress, the Department of Defense (DoD), and the U.S. Department of Veterans Affairs (VA) convened a number of task forces (e.g., Department of Defense Task Force on Mental Health, 2007), commissions, and reviews to highlight major problems and associated solutions, including more resources, policy changes, and stepped-up assessment of efforts to improve care for psychological health problems and traumatic brain injuries (TBI). As part of these efforts, there has been increasing attention on the importance of enhancing psychological resilience (the process of coping with or overcoming exposure to adversity or stress [Wald et al., 2006]) and developing programs to support the military community to increase resilience in light of ongoing deployments.

Psychological resilience is seen as an important component of duty fitness because the operational tempo associated with the conflicts in Iraq and Afghanistan has been demanding for U.S. service members and their families. Service members who are deploying for extended periods on a repeated basis face risks associated with combat that may challenge individuals' and families' coping resources. While most military personnel and their families report coping successfully under these difficult circumstances, many also experience difficulties handling stress at some point. There are, however, programs and strategies available to promote and support psychological resilience to stress—specifically deployment-related stress. An important distinction between approaches to promote resilience, as compared with traditional medical interventions, is the emphasis on prevention as opposed to treatment.

The research on psychological resilience has not been in a form that can be used easily by the military to identify which factors are informed by scientific evidence.

Most of the research on factors that promote resilience has been conducted with community-based and school-based interventions that have been developed in both the military and in other settings to teach resilience skills to individuals and families. While some of these programs have been widely disseminated and shown by research to be effective—such as the Army's Battlemind program (Adler et al., 2009a, and Adler et al., 2009b)[1]—by and large, there is little evidence for whether most programs truly build resilience.

To assist DoD in understanding evidence-informed practices and methodologies useful in promoting psychological resilience in service members and their families, RAND's National Defense Research Institute (RAND NDRI) conducted a literature review of evidence-informed practices for promoting psychological resilience and reviewed a subset of existing programs to determine the extent to which they reflect those evidence-informed practices. In the following sections, we provide a brief summary of the origins of psychological resilience research, how these principles apply to the military, and how resilience programs are beginning to incorporate these principles. We conclude the chapter with a description of our study objectives, our data collection steps, and an outline of the rest of the monograph.

What Is Resilience?

The term *resilience* initially came from the field of engineering with regard to the physical strength of material. *Merriam-Webster's* definition of resilience in the engineering sense is "the capability of a strained body to recover its size and shape after deformation caused especially by compressive stress." Resilience is also defined by *Merriam-Webster* in the psychological sense as "an ability to recover from or adjust easily to misfortune or change."

Psychological Resilience

The idea of physical resilience was extrapolated to psychological resilience and has been defined in a number of ways by several scholars in this broad-ranging field. Despite the lack of universal acceptance of a definition for psychological resilience (Wald et al., 2006), many definitions share some common attributes, including strength to endure some type of traumatic stress or adverse circumstances. Some definitions focus on adaptive coping that results in coming back to baseline functioning levels, while others emphasize positive growth (Connor, 2006; Punamaki et al., 2006; Tedeschi and Calhoun, 2003; and Tedeschi and Calhoun, 2004) or thriving and flourishing (Fredrickson et al., 2003) beyond baseline functioning.

The concept of psychological resilience is rooted in a number of fields. It originated, in large part, in developmental psychology and childhood psychopathology in the 1970s as a result of research showing that despite being raised in extreme poverty

---

[1]   The Army recently changed the name of the Battlemind program to Resiliency Training.

and other adverse circumstances, some children had surprisingly normal developmental trajectories (Bonanno and Mancini, 2008; Garmezy, 1991; and Werner, 1995). The trauma literature also embraced resilience as a construct, with attention to differences in resilience between children and adults as well as between chronic and acute stressors (Bonanno, 2004; Bonanno and Mancini, 2008; and Rachman, 1978). The literature on community resilience suggests that resilience can be built in the wake of school and workplace violence by having credible authorities explain what happened and discuss common reactions to crisis (Nucifora, 2007) or through coping strategies to facilitate problem solving to prevent or alleviate the negative emotional consequences of stressful life circumstances (Ano and Vasconcelles, 2005).

The positive psychology movement (Seligman and Csikszentmihalyi, 2000) also placed more emphasis on psychological resilience, with a shift in focus from what makes people psychologically ill to what keeps people psychologically healthy. Positive psychology focuses on three qualities: positive emotions, positive individual traits, and positive institutions. Martin Seligman's Positive Psychology Center defines positive emotions to include contentment with the past, happiness in the present, and hope for the future (Fredrickson et al., 2003). Individual traits involve strengths and virtues, including the capacity for love and work, courage, compassion, resilience, creativity, curiosity, integrity, self-knowledge, moderation, self-control, and wisdom. The idea of positive institutions encapsulates the study of the strengths that foster better communities, such as justice, responsibility, civility, parenting, nurturance, work ethic, leadership, teamwork, purpose, and tolerance.

Psychological resilience typically goes beyond individual personality traits. It is a process that involves interaction between an individual, his or her past experiences, and current life context (Lepore and Revenson, 2006). Luthar et al. (2000) notes that there are still discrepancies about different conceptualizations of resilience as a personal trait versus a dynamic process. Masten (1994) has recommended that the term *resilience* be reserved to describe the process of adjustment after experiencing significant adversity. This recommendation is based on the concern that labeling an individual as having or lacking the personality trait of resilience carries the risk that some people will feel that they have inadequate resources for coping. Thus, based on this literature, we consider competence despite adversity as resilience, whereas resiliency is considered a trait. We focus our study on the process of resilience. We also consider resilience to be a process, because if it were a trait, it would not be malleable; therefore, training to improve resilience would be futile.

For the purposes of this study, we use the following definition, while acknowledging the lack of consensus around a single definition:

> "Resilience is the capacity to adapt successfully in the presence of risk and adversity" (Jensen and Fraser, 2005).

We chose this definition for several reasons. First, it encapsulates the concept of capacity and the concept of a process involving adaptation and experiencing stressful situations. Also, consistent with the literature, it lends itself to conceptualizing outcomes in a positive orientation (psychological health and strength) rather than a negative one (mental illness and weakness) (Luthar et al., 2000). This definition is also consistent with many of the definitions found in our review (see Chapter Three) and is parsimonious while at the same time is flexible across contexts (e.g., it can be applied to combat as well as poverty).

Framework for Factors That Promote Resilience

Figure 1.1 illustrates the framework we employed to organize the resilience factors by the level of conceptual focus. We used such an organizing framework to distinguish intrinsic factors that promote resilience within an individual from resilience factors that involve other individuals who are part of a group (e.g., family, organization, community). This approach emphasizes transaction and integrative perspectives (Bronfenbrenner, 1977, and Cicchetti and Lynch, 1993) in depicting how resilience factors operate at different levels of the military environment, from the individual level to the broader community level.[2] Our focus in searching the literature was on nonstatic factors associated with psychological resilience. Therefore, we intentionally excluded demographic characteristics and personality traits that would not be changeable as a result of intervention. We reviewed the literature for evidence-informed factors that can be changed. The specific types of resilience factors identified for each level are described in Chapter Three.

How Does Resilience Apply to the Military?

Psychological resilience is important for the military community with regard to keeping military members and leaders fit for duty and to protecting the health and well-being of military families. This monograph focuses on understanding resilience factors and programs designed to promote resilience within the military context. A resilience approach is particularly salient for military culture because it may address the ever-present concerns about the stigma of needing help for psychological or behavioral problems. Despite recent changes in DoD policy, some service members still do not enjoy complete confidentiality in seeking help for emotional and behavioral problems.[3]

---

[2] While resilience factors may broadly operate as being nested within layers moving outward from the individual toward group levels, the specific levels that are most salient will vary across individuals. For example, single service members may view the unit as being more important than factors at the family level, compared with married service members. Accordingly, spouses of reservists may place more primacy on factors that operate at the community level, as compared with the unit level.

[3] In the spring of 2008, Secretary of Defense Robert M. Gates announced a new policy to reduce mental health stigma. This policy eliminates an obstacle to care for mental health problems by revising the language of Question 21 on Standard Form 86, the government security-clearance form that specifically asks applicants

Figure 1.1
Framework for Factors That Promote Resilience

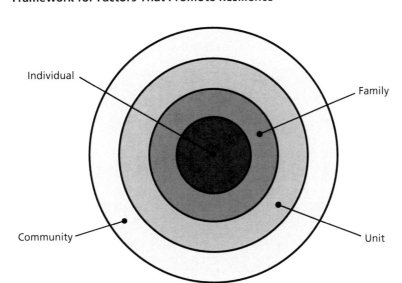

However, leadership can play a pivotal role in creating a command climate in which it is okay to get help for psychological health concerns. Thus, current policy can still promote cultural attitudes and beliefs that inhibit acknowledging problems and seeking mental health care (Tanielian and Jaycox, 2008). While these attitudes and beliefs engender pride, toughness, independence, and self-sufficiency, they can also complicate the task of encouraging service members to seek help for psychological health concerns. Within this context, an emphasis on strengths, such as fitness, thriving, and combating stress, has great potential for helping service personnel without the stigma that is typically associated with seeking help. Further, prevention approaches that emphasize strengths instead of weaknesses are inherently less stigmatizing than traditional treatment-oriented interventions. Thus, the emphasis is on prevention to minimize the need for intervention. Another strong value in military culture is unit cohesion, which helps to improve morale and foster resilience. Service personnel develop close bonds with their comrades or combat "buddies" and through this process provide strength and motivation to get each other through intensive training regimens (National Association of Cognitive-Behavioral Therapists; Helmus and Glenn, 2005).

The resilience concept has been the cornerstone of the Defense Centers of Excellence for Psychological Health and Traumatic Brain Injury (DCoE) Resilience Program, which was created in November 2007 as an effort to shift the culture within the

whether they have ever received treatment for mental health issues. Respondents may now answer "no" if they sought help to deal with their combat stress strictly related to adjustments from service in a military combat environment.

Figure 1.2
DCoE Resilience Continuum

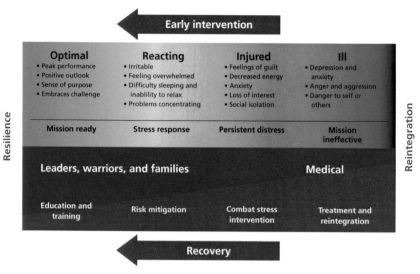

RAND *MG996-1.2*

military away from an illness-focused medical model of care to a model that focuses on psychological health. This emerging model emphasizes "building a culture of resilience" that is driven by respected front line and medical leaders working in partnership to enhance operational readiness for service members and their families. This continuum (Figure 1.2, [DCoE]) was conceived by the Marine Corps and adopted by the DCoE to depict the processes of resilience and reintegration as involving early intervention (in order to maintain resilience) and recovery (in order to return to resilience upon reintegration). A key feature of this continuum is the encapsulation of levels of functioning (from optimal through ill), the intersection of different audiences for targeting interventions (leaders, warriors, families, and medical personnel), and the continuum of interventions tied to restored functioning. This model integrates the following points: (1) psychological health and fitness is just as important as physical health, (2) the system "pushes to the left" across the continuum of optimal, reacting, injured, and ill functional states and supported resilience in every stage of this effort, (3) leaders and front line support agencies play a key role in resilience-building measures, (4) service members and unit leaders (with support from medical) have the greatest involvement in optimizing mission-ready state, maintaining this state when faced with challenges and stressors, and developing strategies that allow individuals and units to return to mission-ready state if they begin to react, (5) the responsibility and involvement of medical personnel increases as service members shift to the right of a mission-ready state, (6) recovery (shifting back to the mission-ready state) is facilitated, encouraged, and promoted from every point on the continuum through extensive supportive elements from community, unit/leadership, family, and personal growth. For most people in the military, prevention and early intervention through education and training will keep them at optimal functioning. Some who show reactions to stress and trauma may need risk mitigation. A smaller number will suffer from distress and need more intensive psychological intervention to help them recover and be reintegrated with their unit. Resilience programs are designed to keep warriors, leaders, and families of the military psychologically fit for duty across the phases of deployment (predeployment, in theater, and post-deployment). It should be noted that the DCoE is currently in the process of updating the continuum model, based on new findings and experience gained while using the present version.

How Is the Military Trying to Promote Psychological Resilience?

As noted, the DoD and the military services have embraced the idea of fostering resilience to maintain a healthy fighting force during wartime. The literature is replete with strategies for promoting resilience in children and families, disaster relief workers and first responders, organizational and community leaders, and, more recently, service members and their families. For example, Wiens and Boss (2006) discusses strategies relevant to military families coping with separation, including deployment preparation for the entire family, employing a "family buddy" analogous to a "battle buddy," unit-level support groups across the phases of deployment, and attention to reunion issues. There are examples of strategies for use in other circumstances as well. These include approaches for keeping individuals, families, and other groups (such as communities) resilient despite poverty, violence, natural disaster, terrorism, and combat. The approaches being used range from single-session group educational counseling to clinician-led treatment interventions (cognitive therapy). However, the clinical treatment interventions are generally reserved for situations in which individuals have not adapted well to adversity. Therefore, these resilience strategies align more closely with prevention than with treatment.

Based on the social science literature, the importance of resilience in the military, and the work by the DCoE to consider these principles, we developed Figure 1.3 to organize this study. The study began with the literature search for the specific types of individual-, family-, unit-,[4] and community-level factors that are based on evidence (left box). These evidence-informed factors are the core features that promote resilience (middle box). Programs that attempt to promote resilience use a number of outcomes to determine whether they are successful (right box). In reviewing selected programs, we sought to understand how these factors are employed to promote resilience, which, in turn, leads to positive outcomes. Positive outcomes can be operationalized using measures of resilience, such as the Conner-Davidson Resilience Scale (CD-RISC) (Connor and Davidson, 2003), or by influencing other types of outcomes, including

---

[4]   We use the term "unit" broadly to include a military work group as well as other types of teams or groups organized for some other purpose (e.g., a corporate committee or work team).

Figure 1.3
Organizing Framework for Promoting Resilience in the Military

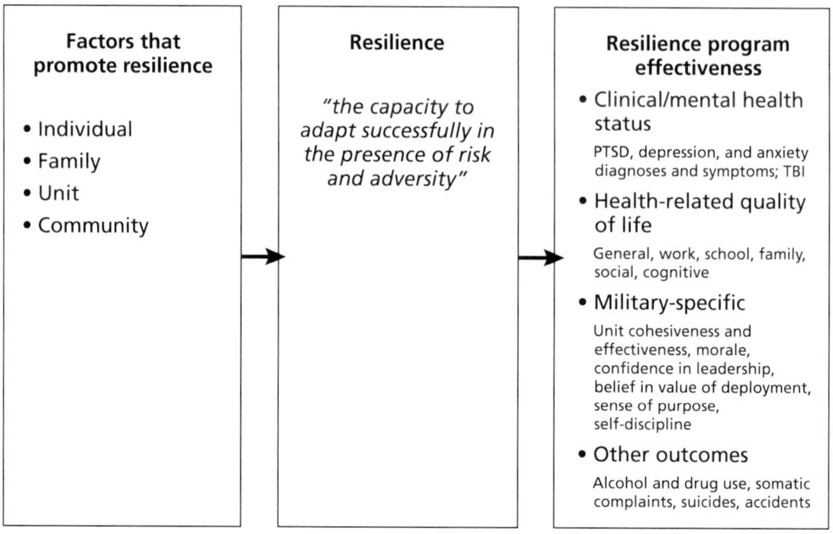

Factors that promote resilience	Resilience	Resilience program effectiveness
• Individual • Family • Unit • Community	*"the capacity to adapt successfully in the presence of risk and adversity"*	• Clinical/mental health status PTSD, depression, and anxiety diagnoses and symptoms; TBI • Health-related quality of life General, work, school, family, social, cognitive • Military-specific Unit cohesiveness and effectiveness, morale, confidence in leadership, belief in value of deployment, sense of purpose, self-discipline • Other outcomes Alcohol and drug use, somatic complaints, suicides, accidents

RAND *MG996-1.3*

clinical, quality of life, and military-specific measures. These outcomes can be used to evaluate the effectiveness of programs that promote resilience.

What Is a Resilience Program?

In addition to defining resilience for this monograph, we have developed a definition for what constitutes a resilience program. This is particularly important because of the rapid proliferation of varying programs emphasizing different strategies and approaches for different target audiences.

For the purpose of this monograph, we define a resilience program as one that targets any of the factors that research has shown to improve resilience and healthy responses to stress, and provides a means for helping individuals to incorporate resilience factors into their daily lives. This definition emphasizes two key rules. First, that programs are based on at least one of the 20 resilience factors identified in the literature review as having some empirical support (these factors were also validated by academic experts in the field of resilience and are listed in Chapter Three). Our definition also specifies that a resilience program enables individuals to use principles and strategies that are informed by scientific evidence.

Research Objectives and Study Approach

Given the need for a systematic analysis of how current military programs are addressing resilience and how well they are incorporating resilience-promoting factors, we sought to address three overarching research objectives. These objectives are listed below with corresponding strategies for accomplishing each. Chapters Two, Three, and Four address each objective in sequence.

- **Objective 1:** Review the literature on psychological resilience with a focus on identifying evidence-informed factors for promoting resilience.
  - To accomplish this objective, we conducted a systematic search and critical review of literature to identify potential evidence-informed factors for promoting resilience. As part of this review, we developed a working definition of resilience that draws on the diverse literatures in psychology, sociology, and medicine to guide the remainder of the project. We also obtained expert input on potential evidence-informed factors from a panel of resilience experts.
- **Objective 2:** Identify and assess current programs relevant to DoD to determine the extent to which they incorporate these evidence-informed factors.
  - Our approach to addressing this objective involved identifying resilience programs and interviewing program staff to assess the extent to which programs included factors that promote resilience. We synthesized interview data with other information obtained about programs to identify themes and assess consistency with the research evidence.
- **Objective 3:** Provide recommendations for future programming or improvements to existing programs that focus on factors that promote resilience.

Organization of This Monograph

This monograph is organized around four chapters. This first chapter describes the study purpose, provides contextual background, and provides an overview of the analytic approach we took in addressing the study objectives. Chapter Two presents the approach and findings from the literature review. Chapter Three presents the approach and findings of our review of resilience programs. Finally, Chapter Four presents conclusions and makes recommendations for improving existing resilience programs and for developing new programs that promote resilience, along with outcome metrics. The appendixes provide definitions of resilience from the literature, a full database of the literature used in the study, and additional information on the resilience programs.

CHAPTER TWO

Literature and Expert Review to Identify Factors That Promote Resilience

In this chapter, we discuss the approach taken and findings from the literature review on factors associated with psychological resilience.[1] We first present the data describing the numbers and types of documents reviewed. We follow with data on evidence ratings for the initial list of resilience factors and then present what we found in the literature, organized by each of the final factors.

Approach

Literature Search

As the first stage of our study,[2] we conducted a review of literature to identify evidence-informed strategies for promoting psychological resilience to stress. We employed a primary database search that covered the literature from January 1, 2000, up to March 20, 2009. After this primary search, we also conducted a secondary search that involved hand-searching the reference lists provided in key literature review articles and book chapters. We also augmented the literature database with documents provided by the DCoE staff and any documents that were provided by program contacts through the program review process that occurred later in the study.

Search Parameters. Our primary search included identifying peer-reviewed citations from the Defense Technical Information Center (DTIC) Private Scientific and

---

[1] Our goal was to identify and describe the various factors that were contained in the literature, based on a qualitative analysis of the available studies. We did not make an attempt to determine how these factors align or are consistent across studies or programs. As such, the factors should be considered an organizing structure that reflects the literature. A principle component factor analysis of the variance, broadly termed "resilience," would be a logical next step. Such an approach would involve scoring the variety of variables, which we've termed "factors," that the literature claims to be enhancers of resilience. Using this method, empirically derived factors, based on clusters of related variance, could be combined and weighted to understand how resilience is actually strengthened or enhanced. Even this strategy, however, would require a degree of researcher judgment, not only for defining the scoring scheme for the factored variables, but also for interpreting the resulting factors or components.

[2] The study protocol was reviewed by the institutional review boards (IRBs) at both RAND and the DoD. RAND approved the study with exempt status (i.e., research that is exempt from ethical review because the only involvement of human subjects falls within certain categories) on December 16, 2008. The TRICARE Management Activity also conducted a second level review of our protocol and also approved the study as exempt on January 23, 2009.

Technical Network (STI-Net), as well as a comprehensive search of peer-reviewed literature (books, articles, reports) from standard databases. DTIC searches utilized the key words (resilience OR resiliency OR resilient) AND (PTSD OR trauma OR stress OR soldier(s) OR veteran(s) OR combat).

The standard database search included PubMed, PsychInfo, PsychArticles, SAGE, OCLC/FirstSearch, Proquest, Web of Science, and Ovid (including CINAHL, Eric, Wiley Science, Google Scholar, and RAND publications). We also searched specific journals, such as the *Journal of Personality and Social Psychology*, the *Journal of Interpersonal Violence*, the *Journal of Family Therapy*, and the *Journal of Clinical Psychology*. Search terms included (resilience OR resiliency OR resilient) AND (PTSD OR intervention OR program(s) OR treatment OR veteran(s) OR soldier(s)).

Exclusion criteria included documents published prior to January 1, 2000,[3] because most of the resilience literature relevant to the military was generated in response to the September 11, 2001, terrorist attacks; documents lacking scientific methods to derive empirical findings; personal narrative or editorials; and documents not in English.

Coding and Data Analysis. Our coding was designed to characterize the documents in three ways:

1. document type (randomized controlled trial (RCT), observational study, theoretical piece, review, or program description)
2. resilience domain (individual, family, unit, or community)
3. body of literature (military mental health, disaster mental health, community violence, or other).

Categories were not considered to be mutually exclusive. We also flagged any definitions of resilience presented in the documents. Most important, we identified factors or program elements that were found to promote resilience.

After the initial document screening for relevance, documents were randomly distributed among five reviewers. Each reviewer completed an abstraction form (available from the authors on request) that included identifying information (number, author[s], and date of publication), instructions for entering the coding information as guided by the criteria above, and an area to indicate if the document should be excluded from the review. We excluded documents either because they provided no information about psychological factors that promote resilience or because the factors discussed were the wrong kind for our study—static and nonmalleable factors, such as demographic characteristics or personality traits. Specifically, we excluded gender, age, race/ethnicity, and marital status, recognizing that while these characteristics may be useful for targeting interventions, these are preexisting factors that cannot be altered by training

---

[3] We limited our selection of articles to those published after January 1, 2000, in our primary search only. We included 18 articles published before this date in the secondary search because we felt that they were particularly relevant to the study.

as part of a resilience program. We also excluded personality traits that, based on the literature, are known to be generally stable. For example, resilience training cannot improve intelligence (including AFQT scores). We also chose to exclude hardiness (Kobasa and Maddi, 1977) because it is traditionally defined as a stable personality trait, even though there is some recent evidence that hardiness training can increase hardiness scores and affect performance under stressful conditions (Maddi et al., 2009; Judkins et al., 2006; Zach et al., 2007). The abstraction form also included an area in which to note specific factors that promote resilience as discussed in the document, any resilience definitions mentioned, empirical evidence provided, and any concerns or limitations of the sample, design, analysis, or findings. All documents were entered into an EndNote database for cataloguing and an Excel database for collecting and analyzing the coded information.

After the documents were reviewed, the research team generated a list of factors identified as promoting or related to resilience using a pile-sort method (Lincoln and Guba, 1985, and Ryan and Bernard, 2003). Each factor that appeared in the Excel database was printed on an individual slip of paper. Four members of the research team reviewed a portion of the slips and sorted them into piles representing similar themes. The team then reviewed and discussed each pile of factors over a series of meetings until all factors were discussed and the team was in agreement about the grouping and final list of factors. Our coding process identified 18 factors in four categories. Five of the 18 factors were aspects of resilience that are at the individual level, five were at the family level, five were at the unit level, and three were at community level. These data are listed in Table 2.1.

Evidence Rating. After the documents were coded, three members of the research team revisited the documents and assigned each document a rating for the strength of scientific evidence to establish causal relationships involving resilience. Raters used the following rating categories:

- **None**—The factor has not been subjected to scientific study. Documents that provided only theoretical explications with no empirical support were assigned this rating.
- **Weak**—The factor has been studied, but there is only minimal or inconclusive evidence. Documents that provided some evidence through weak designs, such as case studies or review articles that cited secondary studies but without details that could be scrutinized, were assigned this rating.
- **Moderate**—The factor has been studied, and there is clear and consistent evidence based on correlational or cross-sectional observational analysis. Documents that provided this level of evidence on a factor were assigned this rating.
- **Strong**—The factor has been studied, and there is clear and consistent evidence based on RCT or longitudinal analysis. Only documents that provided evidence at this rigorous level were assigned this rating.

Table 2.1
Number of Documents at Each Level of Evidence for Each Factor

Factor	Evidence Rating				
	None	Weak	Moderate	Strong	Total
Individual					
Positive coping	3	20	38	2	63
Positive affect	0	13	28	8	49
Positive thinking	1	34	37	6	78
Realism	2	17	29	0	48
Behavioral control	0	9	18	0	27
Family					
Emotional ties	0	5	6	0	11
Communication	0	10	9	0	19
Support	1	12	17	2	32
Closeness	0	4	3	1	8
Nurturing	0	9	10	0	19
Unit					
Positive command climate	1	13	9	0	23
Teamwork	0	5	2	0	7
Reduced stigma	0	0	1	0	1
Unit cohesion	0	11	5	0	16
Role modeling	0	1	1	0	2
Community					
Belongingness	0	30	32	1	63
Connectedness	1	13	7	0	21
Shared values	0	3	2	0	5
Total	9	209	254	20	492

NOTE: A single document may contribute information on more than one factor.

The researchers discussed and reviewed their ratings for each category. A consensus process was used to resolve inconsistencies and reach agreement across raters.

Expert Review

We invited 11 academic experts to vet our initial list of 18 evidence-informed factors that promote resilience. Expert panelists were selected by the team in collaboration with the client. The panelists were chosen because they conduct research on resilience. Panelists received a one-page project description and a two-page rating form. We asked those who agreed to participate to complete a form for rating the 18 factors. The pre-teleconference rating form (available on request) described the study and provided instructions on how to complete it. Panelists were asked to rate each of the factors on three separate 5-point scales in which 5 was the highest rating:

1. importance for promoting resilience
2. difficulty to implement as a resilience program element
3. overall desirability of the resilience factor to be incorporated into a resilience program.

Eight of the 11 invited experts agreed to complete the rating form; some also provided written comments. Seven of these eight experts participated in the 1.5-hour post-rating expert panel phone discussion. We aggregated the expert ratings and provided this information back to the group, along with the agenda and other pertinent information, prior to the phone discussion. The call began with a review of what we did for the literature review phase of the study. Following brief introductions, the summary rating data were reviewed along with the rules of the panel process. The remainder of the time was devoted to discussing points of departure and issues that arose from their comments.

For the rating of "importance for promoting resilience," family support, positive thinking, positive coping, and positive command climate were rated as being the most important. However, there was little variation across the factors (only one scored slightly less than 4 on the 1–5 scale) suggesting that the group generally agreed that the 18 initial factors are all important. Community connectedness, family closeness, social integration, and positive affect were rated highest on "difficulty to implement as a resilience program element." There was more variation on this rating across the factors, with three rated below 3 on the 1–5 scale: teamwork, positive thinking, and positive coping. For "overall desirability of the resilience factor to be incorporated into a resilience program," family support, positive thinking, positive coping, and positive command climate are all rated the highest, and, as with importance, there was little variation across factors (only one was rated below a 4).

Following the teleconference, the research team revised the list of factors according to the panel feedback and sent a summary of the call along with that list back to them for a final review and any additional comments. Table 2.2 shows the final list of 20 factors based on the literature review, alongside the initial list of 18 factors.

Table 2.2
Factors That Promote Resilience from Literature Review: Before and After Expert Review

Level	Factors Before Expert Review (n=18)	Factors After Expert Review (n=20)
Individual	Coping, positive affect, positive thinking, realism, behavioral control	**Positive** coping, positive affect, positive thinking, realism, behavioral control, **physical fitness, altruism**
Family	Emotional ties, communication, support, closeness, nurturing	Emotional ties, communication, support, closeness, nurturing, **adaptability**
Unit	Positive command climate, teamwork, **reduced stigma, unit** cohesion, **role modeling**	Positive command climate, teamwork, cohesion
Community	Belongingness, connectedness, **shared values**	Belongingness, **cohesion**, connectedness, collective efficacy

NOTE: Changes based on experts are shown in bold in the Before column if dropped and in the After column if added or relabeled.

Findings

Literature Search

We screened a total of 340 documents using a two-stage process: First, the titles and abstracts of articles were screened to determine if they addressed the general topic; then, the subset of screened documents was coded using an abstraction form. Of the 340 documents screened, 137 were from the primary database search, and 203 were found through hand searches of review articles or chapters and other sources.[4] After dropping documents that did not meet the initial screening criteria (25 from the primary search and 45 from the secondary search) for the study, we identified 270 documents to review (112 primary and 158 secondary). All 270 documents are listed in Appendix B.1. Of those reviewed, 187 were retained for coding (75 primary and 112 secondary) because they contributed information about at least one resilience factor (i.e., 83 were rejected after review). Figure 2.1 summarizes this information.

Identifying the Factors. After coding, 149 documents contributed information about factors that promote resilience. Coders identified factors that promote resilience as they reviewed each document. For coding purposes, a factor was defined as a theoretical concept or measurable construct that can be taught or practiced and was described or demonstrated to be associated with resilience and/or outcomes of resilience. Of the documents we reviewed, the majority were either review articles (*n*=79) or observational studies (*n*=75). We identified very few that were controlled trials (*n*=11). The bulk of the documents examined individual-level resilience (*n*=143), though family

---

[4]   Hand search involved a "snowball" approach in which the research team reviewed the reference lists of other articles and book chapters, primarily review documents, to identify those that met our inclusion criteria.

Figure 2.1
Literature Search Results

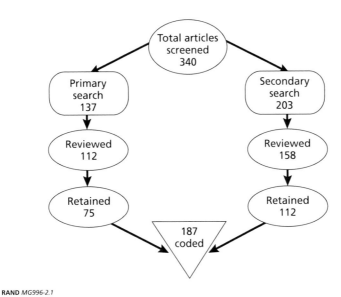

(n=41), unit (n=23), and community-level factors (n=25) were also addressed. Most of the literature was found in the military mental health area (n=72), and another large group was from the general psychology field (n=106).

Rating the Factors. Prior to the expert panel, we had identified 18 different factors from the literature review, as listed in Table 2.1, which summarizes the evidence ratings for each. Because more than one factor could have been included in each document, the numbers add to more than the total number of documents. The bulk of the ratings across the different factors were either weak (209 documents) or moderate (254 documents). As expected, few were rated as having no evidence (9 documents), in part because we had already identified most of the documents as contributing information about a factor. Only 13 documents were rated as having strong evidence for at least one factor.[5] There was stronger evidence pertaining to individual factors that promote resilience (especially positive coping, positive affect, positive thinking, and realism), with family support the next strongest. Unit-level factors had less evidence relative to the other factors, though positive command climate had the most evidence within that level. Among the community-level factors, social integration had a good deal of evidence for promoting resilience. These data are also summarized in Figure 2.2, which shows the relative levels of evidence in terms of percentage within each category. Of note is the fact that only one document contributed evidence for reduced stigma.

---

[5] Some of the documents provide evidence for more than one factor; these are listed in Chapter Two.

Figure 2.2
Aggregate Scores—Strength of Factor Evidence

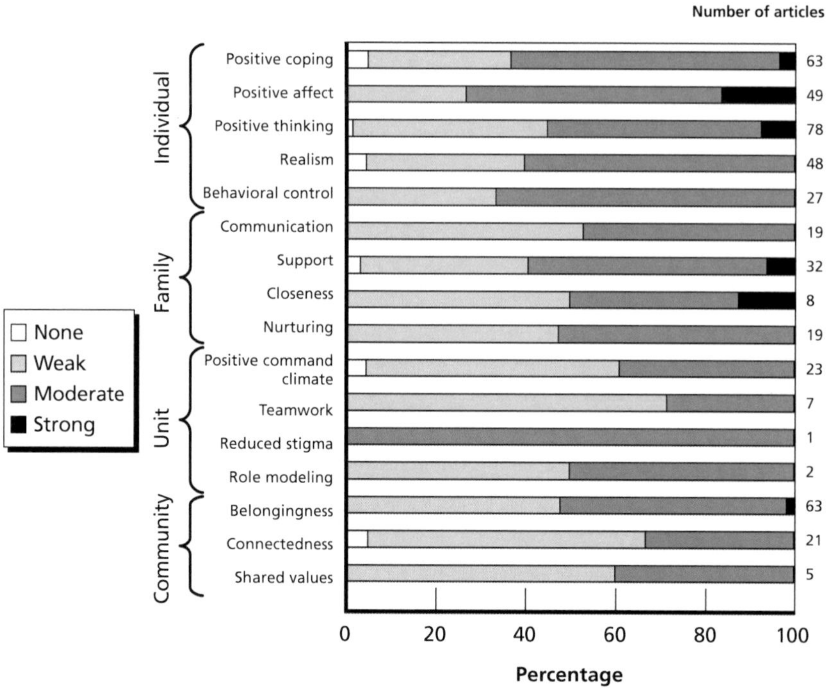

RAND *MG996-2.2*

Expert Panel. Based on our ratings, we changed several of the factors before we presented them to the expert panel.[6] We dropped reduced stigma, given that there was only one document contributing evidence, and incorporated role modeling into the positive command climate factor from the unit-level list. We also renamed emotion regulation as behavioral control to distinguish it from positive affect, which captured the emotional content. Finally, we revised the community resilience factors by merging shared values with connectedness and relabeling social integration as social capital (later renamed belongingness by a reviewer), which still includes integration. These changes resulted in an updated list of 18 factors. This list was shared with the expert panel. The expert panelists recommended that two additional individual factors be added to the list. One was physical fitness, which was not included in our literature review focused on psychological factors. Nevertheless, it was regarded by the panel to be important for the military culture. The other was altruism.

In terms of the ratings, there was little variation across the eight experts with regard to "importance for promoting resilience." Ratings for all of the 16 resilience

---

[6]   Some of the factor labels were also changed after the expert panel. As we explored particular programs and considered their content and the policy implications of our findings, we realized that there were ways to characterize the factors in ways that provided greater clarity and practical utility.

components were mostly fours and fives with a few three-point ratings on the five-point scale. Positive command climate, family support, positive thinking, and realism were at the top of the list in terms of importance, but, again, all were deemed important. In contrast, group ratings for "difficulty to implement as a resilience program element" varied widely across the different components. For several of the individual, family, and unit-level factors, ratings ranged more than three points on the five-point scale. For example, one person rated family support a one while another rated it a five, with others rating this factor somewhere between one and five. Communication, positive thinking, positive coping, and teamwork were viewed as being least difficult to incorporate into a resilience program. The ratings for "overall desirability of the resilience factor/element to be incorporated into a resilience program" mirrored the data for "importance," with essentially the same factors rated the highest. Again, as with importance, there was little variation, with only one factor rated below a four (collective efficacy).

The panelists also made some comments about the framework and factors more broadly. Overall, the group thought that the list of factors and framework was appropriate, but they suggested some ways to clarify and improve on that initial list. For example, they liked the multiple system levels and thought that the family and unit categories were very clear but that the individual and community sections could be clearer. Some of the constructs needed to be better defined operationally (e.g., realism). They also suggested that pragmatism should be included as part of positive coping to address the distinction between positive thinking and cognitive style. It was also noted among the group that the "difficulty" rating was hard to determine because it was not clear whether it applied to measurement of the component or to training/teaching the component (which could explain the greater variation in ratings).

There was extensive discussion about overlap across the constructs, particularly for positive thinking, realism, and coping, as well as cohesion and connectedness. The expert panelists determined that connectedness is about connection to place or people of a place, and cohesion is more about shared values or emotional ties. The group also agreed that hope should be included in the positive affect factor and that institutional policy should be included under positive command climate and belongingness.

The expert panelists cautioned against using the term *resilience* to refer to something substantive that can be taught in and of itself. Instead, they suggested that we use the term to describe response to a stressful experience. In other words, efforts should not try to define resilience per se but instead focus on the factors contributing to resilience. This is, in fact, the approach that RAND took. A general concern among expert panelists was that many resilience programs are offered to DoD by outside contractors with no evidence for success. They also emphasized that resilience may change over time and that different components may be important for each domain—one can be resilient in one context but not another.

The expert panel also suggested adding altruism as an individual resilience factor because it is a crucial aspect of the sacrifice of military service and is also associated with reductions in grief and survivor guilt. In addition, the panel suggested adding another factor for family-level resilience—adaptability. Finally, the panel recommended that cohesion be pulled out as a separate factor within community-level resilience, due to the consensus on the definition. These changes resulted in a final list of 20 evidence-informed factors.

General Findings from the Literature Review

In this section, we first present information on the various definitions of resilience that we found in the 187 coded documents. We then present data on the factors that were identified in the 149 documents contributing some evidence for at least one of the 20 final resilience factors. In this section, we refer to supporting literature using the document numbers that map to the EndNote database used for this study, listed in Appendix B.2.

Definitions of Resilience. As we reviewed each document in our literature review, we also tracked the various definitions of resilience described. In some cases, these definitions may have originated in previous documents, and some documents listed multiple definitions. For example, Norris et al. (2008) provides a table of various definitions for community resilience, and Luthar et al. (2000) provides a critical analysis of the resilience construct, including a discussion about the varying types of definitions. However, our purpose was to get a sense of the types of definitions and the extent to which they appear in the documents about factors that promote resilience. We classified the definitions we found along a continuum of three main types of definitions:

1. **basic**—definitions that describe resilience as a process or capacity that develops over time
2. **adaptation**—definitions that incorporate the concept of "bouncing back," adapting, or returning to a baseline after experiencing adversity or trauma
3. **growth**—definitions that additionally involve growth after experiencing adversity or trauma.

This classification system is similar to the one used by Masten (1994, 1990). Based on our literature review, we identified 122 definitions, which are summarized in Appendix A along with their sources. We chose to use the most common type of definition, which emphasizes adaptation. A few definitions of resilience centered around capacity without explicitly including the concept of adaptation or "bouncing back" ($n=24$), such as examples provided by Mancini and Bonanno (2006) and Letourneau et al. (2001). Most of the definitions found in the literature that we reviewed did emphasize adaptation ($n=80$), such as examples from Fredrickson et al. (2003) and Jensen and Fraser (2005). Some of the definitions went further by specifying the concept of improving or growth following adversity ($n=18$), such as examples from Connor

(2006) and Punamaki et al. (2006). Eighteen of the definitions were about community resilience (Appendix A.2).

Factors That Promote Resilience. Table 2.3 provides the factors by level, along with the operational definitions. The definitions were crafted based on definitions found in the literature and were supplemented by comments made by the expert panelists.

Table 2.3
Summary of Final Evidence-Informed Resilience Factors That Promote Resilience

Resilience Factors	Operational Definition
Individual Level	
Positive coping	The process of managing taxing circumstances, expending effort to solve personal and interpersonal problems, and seeking help to reduce or tolerate stress or conflict, including active/pragmatic, problem-focused, and spiritual approaches to coping
Positive affect	Feeling enthusiastic, active, and alert, including having positive emotions, optimism, a sense of humor (ability to have humor under stress or when challenged), hope, and flexibility about change
Positive thinking	Information processing, applying knowledge, and changing preferences through restructuring, positive reframing, making sense out of a situation, flexibility, reappraisal, refocusing, having positive outcome expectations, a positive outlook, and psychological preparation
Realism	Realistic mastery of the possible/having realistic outcome expectations, self-esteem/self-worth, confidence, self-efficacy, perceived control/acceptance of what is beyond control or cannot be changed
Behavioral control	The process of monitoring, evaluating, and modifying reactions to accomplish a goal (i.e., self-regulation, self-management, self-enhancement)
Physical fitness	Bodily ability to function efficiently and effectively in life domains
Altruism	Selfless concern for the welfare of others, motivation to help without reward
Family Level	
Emotional ties	Emotional bonding among family members, including shared recreation and leisure time
Communication	The exchange of thoughts, opinions, or information, including problem-solving and relationship management
Support	Perceiving that comfort is available from (and can be provided to) others, including emotional, tangible, instrumental, informational, and spiritual support
Closeness	Love, intimacy and attachment
Nurturing	Parenting skills
Adaptability	Ease of adapting to changes associated with military life, including flexible roles within the family

Table 2.3—Continued

Resilience Factors	Operational Definition
Unit Level	
Positive command climate	Facilitating and fostering intra-unit interaction, building pride/support for the mission, leadership, positive role modeling, and implementing institutional policies
Teamwork	Work coordination among team members, including flexibility
Cohesion	Team ability to perform combined actions; bonding together of members to sustain commitment to each other and the mission
Community Level	
Belongingness	Integration, friendships; group membership, including participation in spiritual/faith-based organizations, protocols, ceremonies, social services, schools, and so on; and implementing institutional policies
Cohesion	The bonds that bring people together in the community, including shared values and interpersonal belonging
Connectedness	The quality and number of connections with other people in the community; includes connections with a place or people of that place; aspects include commitment, structure, roles, responsibility, and communication
Collective efficacy	Group members' perceptions of the ability of the group to work together

NOTE: Two of the individual-level resilience factors included in the final list of 20, physical fitness and altruism, were not identified from the literature review. Therefore, we did not rate the evidence for them. However, because the expert panelists suggested that they be added, we conducted a post hoc search of our existing literature database and identified a few documents that discussed these as potential resilience factors.

Findings from the Literature Review by Resilience Factor

In the remainder of this section, key findings from the literature reviews are organized by each of the different levels of resilience factors in the organizing framework—from individual through community. The objective is to highlight some of the study findings on how each factor can be employed to promote resilience and improve health and functioning.

Table 2.4 shows the documents (by document number) that, based on the literature review, were determined to contribute either moderate or strong evidence in support of at least one factor for promoting resilience. The table makes it clear that some factors are more researched than others. For example, positive coping, positive affect, positive thinking, realism, behavioral control, family support, and belongingness have many references to evidence. A few of the factors were only minimally supported, including altruism, adaptability, teamwork, community-level cohesion, and collective efficacy. Only 13 documents were rated as having strong evidence in the literature—#2, #223, #248, #254, #263, #272, #277, #293, #295, #330, #344, #345,

Table 2.4
Summary of Evidence-Informed Resilience Factors and Supporting Literature

Resilience Factors	Supporting Literature	
	Moderate Evidence	Strong Evidence
Individual		
Positive coping	2, 3, 21, 30, 45, 62, 98, 118, 149, 152, 155, 164, 166, 169, 172, 178, 191, 195, 201, 216, 230, 245, 246, 254, 271, 274, 277, 292, 294, 295, 314, 321, 325, 329, 332, 343, 353, 354	248, 330
Positive affect	3, 6, 21, 62, 65, 81, 144, 149, 152, 155, 156, 164, 166, 216, 226, 229, 245, 294, 295, 312, 314, 321, 332, 343, 347, 350, 351, 353	2, 254, 263, 272, 277, 344, 345, 346
Positive thinking	2, 3, 51, 62, 65, 144, 145, 149, 152, 155, 156, 159, 164, 166, 169, 174, 188, 201, 218, 226, 229, 245, 246, 271, 288, 294, 295, 305, 314, 315, 321, 326, 332, 340, 350, 351, 353	254, 263, 277, 293, 344, 346
Realism	2, 3, 21, 62, 144, 149, 155, 159, 166, 169, 178, 201, 206, 223, 226, 228, 229, 245, 288, 292, 294, 295, 314, 321, 325, 329, 332, 343, 353	none
Behavioral control	3, 23, 24, 149, 155, 159, 189, 209, 243, 246, 314, 321, 326, 347, 348, 351, 353, 354	none
Family		
Emotional ties	62, 152, 178, 195, 250, 318	none
Communication	152, 159, 169, 240, 243, 278, 318, 321, 351	none
Support	152, 166, 178, 187, 188, 195, 197, 209, 212, 218, 240, 243, 278, 314, 318, 325, 332	223, 248
Closeness	159, 314, 318	none
Nurturing	101, 159, 166, 178, 187, 188, 223, 243, 246, 318	none
Unit		
Positive command climate	31, 148, 218, 240, 271, 272, 283, 305, 317	none
Teamwork	218, 351	none
Cohesion	45, 82, 148, 218, 340	none
Community		
Belongingness	3, 23, 51, 60, 62, 66, 82, 101, 152, 178, 183, 188, 193, 195, 212, 221, 226, 229, 238, 239, 240, 241, 243, 245, 250, 260, 273, 278, 291, 292, 315, 317	295

Table 2.4—Continued

Resilience Factors	Supporting Literature	
	Moderate Evidence	Strong Evidence
Cohesion	20, 169, 252, 280	none
Connectedness	3, 164, 195, 245, 275, 278, 318	none
Collective efficacy	None (245, 252, 268 with weak evidence)	none

NOTE: Entries correspond to the reference numbers in the bibliography. These documents were rated by the research team as having moderate (clear and consistent evidence based on correlational or cross-sectional observational analysis) to strong support (evidence is from a randomized controlled trial or longitudinal analysis) on the basis of information available in the document. Evidence was not rated for adaptability, physical fitness, and altruism, since these factors were added by the experts after the rating process was complete.

and #346. Seven of these provided evidence for more than one resilience factor (#248, #254, #263, #277, #330, #444, and #346).

Individual-Level Factors. From the literature review, we identified seven types of evidence-informed individual-level factors that have been demonstrated to promote resilience. These include positive coping, positive affect, positive thinking, realism, behavioral control, physical fitness, and altruism. These last two factors were added after the literature review, so they are not shown in Table 2.4.

Positive Coping. The literature examining the role of individual positive coping in response to stressful situations indicates that problem-solving approaches are effective in enhancing one's ability to reduce or tolerate stress or conflict. Successful coping techniques may include reappraisals of challenging situations from one of three perspectives: active/pragmatic, problem-focused, or spiritual. For example, an RCT (#2) found that a four-day, 30-hour intensive train-the-trainer course on how to cope with stress predicts how participants handle emotional difficulties. The active use of training (e.g., coping skills, understanding somatic reactions, identifying and clarifying feelings, normalizing fears, coping with grief/loss, turning crisis into opportunity, dealing with anger and rage, seeking a better future) was particularly helpful for teaching disaster survivors to be more resilient. A longitudinal study found that approach-oriented coping (defined as active planning, directly dealing with difficult situations rather than avoiding them, and focusing on the positive) predicted better family and social functioning among patients with PTSD. These findings suggest that, despite having symptoms of PTSD, individuals who use these coping techniques can maintain better relationships (#118). Our review highlighted 63 studies that identified coping as an individual resilience factor. However, the strongest evidence for the role of positive coping as a resilience factor came from two studies. One of these studies used a three-year prospective design with 400 married couples to examine couple resilience to economic pressure (#248). Couples who demonstrated the ability to generate realistic and nonexploitative solutions to their conflicts and disagreements and who resolved their disagreements more quickly were less likely to suffer from marital distress. The other study (#330) used a prospective design with 801 Navy recruits to assess the effects of a boot camp survival-training intervention on stress. This study found that the intervention increased sense of belonging, decreased loneliness, and increased use of problem-solving coping skills; further, these recruits were less likely to transfer or separate from service. Moderate support for this factor came from 38 documents (see Table 2.4).

Positive Affect. Another important individual-level resilience factor is positive affect, which is defined as keeping an optimistic outlook. Approaches that encourage people to maintain hope, keep a positive outlook, or deal with stress by talking and finding humor in situations (where appropriate) help release tension. As an example, one empirical study of 328 Air Force medical personnel (#81) showed that having an optimistic attitude in the face of transient situational demands was associated with greater resilience (assessed with the Connor-Davidson measure, 2003), including the ability to recover from negative and stressful experiences and find positive meaning in seemingly adverse situations. We identified 49 documents with evidence for positive affect as a factor in resilience. These studies have looked at a range of resilience-related outcomes from the role that positive emotions play in increasing capacity for tolerating stress, lowering stress-related illness, decreasing use of health care services, reducing symptoms of depression, and decreasing autonomic arousal (as summarized in #254). Eight of these documents contributed strong evidence, and 28 documents contributed moderate evidence.

Positive Thinking. We identified a number of documents in support of positive thinking techniques to promote resilience. One review cited evidence that training, which emphasizes the development of realistic outcome expectations, is associated with resilience (#218) using a stress risk–management framework. Altogether, there were 78 documents that identified positive thinking techniques that can help people refocus or reframe a situation in a more positive or constructive way, such as making sense out of challenging circumstances. The strongest evidence came from six documents, and moderate evidence came from 37 documents.

Realism. Teaching people how to achieve realism about their situations is another evidence-informed strategy for promoting resilience. One study reported that realism restores people to previous functioning and inspires others to find new meaning in their lives (#288). There were 48 documents in our review that identified realism as a factor in resilience. None of these documents presented strong evidence, but 29 of them had moderate evidence. As an example, the review by Hoge (#62) reported that realism, defined as having an internal locus of control, is protective against stress in children and adolescents. Another study (#3) stated that there is broad empirical support for self-efficacy facilitating positive adaptation following trauma.

Behavioral Control. Self-regulation of behavior also seems to promote resilience. Specifically, behavioral control strategies, such as self-enhancement, have been linked with fewer PTSD and depressive symptoms (#24). According to Masten (2001), studies consistently find a link between self-regulation skills and resilience (#246). We identified 27 documents with evidence for behavioral control. While none of these presented strong evidence, 18 documents had moderate evidence for behavioral control as a resilience strategy. An example in support of behavioral control is that a better understanding of the link between beliefs, feelings, and behavior, a key component of the Penn Resiliency Project (PRP), is associated with reduced depression symptoms in children (#321).

Physical Fitness. As noted earlier, physical fitness was not initially included in our document search, nor was evidence rated for this factor. However, we conducted a post hoc search of our existing literature database and identified four documents that provide support for physical fitness as a beneficial aspect of resilience interventions (#95, #166, #325, and #351, not shown in Table 3.4; see Appendix B).

Altruism. The expert panel also suggested that we add altruism to our list of individual resilience factors, even though the literature review did not identify that specific factor. In a post hoc search, we did find one document that noted the importance of altruism, defined as "selfless acts" including an altruistic outlook toward others (#254). This document suggests that altruism may be associated with resilience, and the selfless acts may increase well-being for promoting resilience. Again, evidence was not rated for this factor.

Family-Level Factors. Because military families are under stress—particularly because deployment separates them—programs that support these factors may enhance resilience and ability to cope with deployment. We identified six family-level resilience factors: emotional ties, communication, support, closeness, nurturing, and adaptability.

Emotional Ties. Emotional ties in parents were associated with resilience in 11 of the documents we identified. For example, nurturing and involved parenting can ease the transitions from childhood to adolescence and from adolescence to early adulthood (#178). None of the documents identified had strong evidence for emotional ties, and only six presented moderate evidence. A study by Black and Lobo (#152) found that "families who play together stay together," as evidenced by lower divorce and separation rates.

Communication. Communication among family members is supported more strongly by the literature—we identified 19 documents with some evidence. We found no documents providing strong supporting evidence, but nine documents provided moderate evidence for communication as a resilience factor. One of them (#243) found that parent communication, including expressions of concern, was positively associated with childhood resilience (defined as future expectations for high school graduation and having a happy family life), especially among victimized children. Specifically, communication increases capacity for children to share and respond to feelings and to better connect with returning service members after lengthy periods away.

Support. Another family-level resilience factor is support, or the perceived emotional, tangible, informational, and spiritual comfort available from and provided to others. Pilot studies have shown that enhanced quality of early interactions between parents and their children (including support for the parents) may reduce mental health difficulties in children and reduce family stress (#187). Another study showed that individual and family coping resources mediate the problems of violence on child outcomes (#197). Thirty-two documents identified family support as a factor in resilience. The strongest evidence came from two documents (#223 and #248). The latter of these two found that high levels of marital support reduced the association between economic stress and emotional distress. Moderate evidence came from 17 documents.

Closeness. Closeness—love, intimacy, and attachment—was identified as a resilience factor in eight documents, but only three provided moderate evidence, and none provided strong evidence. As reported in the review by MacDermid et al. (#159), parental displays of warmth and closeness are linked with the development of resilience in children, particularly if these factors are combined with "reasonable, firm, and consistent limit-setting." A study by Yehuda et al. (#314) reported that love, intimacy, and attachment are associated with psychological well-being and resilience.

Nurturing. Nurturing by way of good parenting skills was one of the family factors with good evidence in the literature for supporting resilience. For example, interventions that include parenting skills reduce family stress (#187), and parent support for the child is related to child resilience (#243). We found 19 studies that identified nurturing as a resilience factor. None of these provided strong support, but ten documents showed moderate evidence.

Adaptability. Having adaptability in family roles is another important resilience factor. For example, maintaining family adaptability has been demonstrated to be a protective factor in families who have children with disabilities (#196). Other documents in our post hoc review that identified adaptability as a resilience factor are #152 and #253. The expert panelists recommended that this factor be separated from positive affect as in the original set of factors after the evidence rating process, and so it was not rated, nor is it shown in Table 2.4.

Unit-Level Factors. The literature also helps us understand the unit-level factors that contribute to resilience. The literature has shown that certain aspects of military life, including strong and positive command climate, teamwork, and unit cohesion, are important for keeping service members resilient (see Table 2.4).

Positive Command Climate. Positive command climate is identified in the literature as contributing to resilience. Leaders can facilitate team-building by emphasizing unique skills and talents of service members in the unit, which in turn can help to build mastery and confidence among troops. We found 23 documents that cited positive command climate as contributing to resilience. While none of these presented strong evidence, nine gave moderate evidence. One study, based on surveys to identify leadership qualities, found that leaders who empower and support their workforces, by helping them appreciate the meaning of their work, enhance a sense of personal control and cohesion (as reviewed in #271). Additionally, leaders can enhance psychological resilience of their team by reinforcing a sense of self-efficacy. Bliese (#283) found that soldiers with leaders who established a positive social climate had better psychological well-being; that well-being, in turn, improved resilience and job satisfaction in combat.

Teamwork. Teamwork, or work coordination and flexibility among team members, was identified in seven documents as related to resilience. None of the documents presented strong evidence for teamwork, but two documents gave moderate evidence. For example, as summarized in a review by Paton (#218), effective teamwork that involves good sharing of information can enhance resilience to stress among police officers during the response and reintegration phases of incident response. Central to this idea is that team members need to share a common mindset that facilitates use of information toward common goals to aid decisions.

Unit Cohesion. Unit cohesion, defined as a military unit's ability to perform combat actions, bond together, and sustain commitment to each other and the mission, is another evidence-based strategy for promoting resilience. We identified five documents as presenting moderate evidence for this factor. None of the documents gave strong evidence for unit cohesion. However, one study found that unit cohesion predicted PTSD symptoms and also attenuated the association between stress and PTSD among soldiers sampled at the battalion-level military unit (#148).

Community-Level Factors. Four different resilience factors were identified at the community level: belongingness, cohesion, group connectedness, and collective efficacy.

Belongingness. Belongingness includes social integration; group membership or participation in spiritual/faith-based organizations, protocols, ceremonies, social services, and schools; and implementation of institutional policies. Belongingness can operate through cultural symbolic structures and systems (such as community spirit that gives members a "secure base") to improve individual development in military members. In one study (#60) belongingness, assessed as "strong community spirit," was associated with low rates of PTSD and high subjective well-being scores. We identified 63 documents with some evidence for belongingness as a resilience factor. Only one document provided strong evidence, but 32 documents provided moderate evidence for belongingness as a resilience factor.

Community Cohesion. Community cohesion is broadly defined as perceptions of mission success and achievement for the community. An example is that environments that promote social cohesion or a sense of community can potentially help build capacity for resilience to disasters based on a surveillance study of first responders (#20). Other documents identified in our post hoc analyses as providing some evidence include #169, #252, and #280, but evidence was not rated for this factor. There is more empirical support for unit-level cohesion, though the theoretical literature includes community-level cohesion as a prominent feature that needs more study.

Connectedness. Connectedness is the quality and number of connections with people and places, including such aspects as commitment, structure, roles, responsibility, and communication. We identified 21 documents that discussed this factor. None of these provided strong support, and seven documents provided moderate support for group connectedness as a resilience factor. This factor awaits further empirical examination, but it is posited to be related to resilience within the context of community violence (#278). For example, individuals who are more connected with the neighborhood may have a stronger foundation for coping with the effects of violence. Thus, connectedness can act as a protective factor.

Collective Efficacy. There was only weak evidence for collective efficacy from three review documents (#245, #252, and #268) identified post hoc. These reviews provide secondary support for the idea that group members' confidence in the group's ability to perform its mission may be associated with resilience. For example, one study (Jex and Bliese, 1999, as cited by #268) suggested that individuals who are members of groups with high collective efficacy are less likely to suffer from work stress.

Summary of Literature and Expert Reviews

The literature provides evidence for several factors associated with resilience. These factors span the individual, family, military unit, and broader community and can be incorporated into programs designed to build a stronger fighting force. Individual factors that lead to resilience have been more frequently and more rigorously studied relative to family-, unit-, and community-level factors. Even among the limited number of randomized controlled studies (#2, #45, #187, #189, #277, #321, #330, #331, #344, #345, and #346), the types of factors that promote resilience and samples (e.g., children, Special Forces, families, parents, college students) vary widely, which makes it difficult to draw broad conclusions. Our findings suggest that a number of factors are particularly important for expanding our understanding of military resilience. However, they are understudied and warrant further examination.

CHAPTER THREE

Review of Programs for Promoting Resilience

This chapter describes the approach we used to identify, select, and review resilience programs. We also report the findings from our assessment of a subgroup of resilience programs presented below and organized around four topics:

1. program characteristics
2. strategies for promoting resilience
3. barriers to program implementation
4. evaluation of program effectiveness, including outcome measures used.

Approach

The final phase of the project involved reviewing a set of resilience programs via interviews with program representatives. The purpose of the interviews was to find out to what extent the evidence-informed resilience factors identified in the literature map onto program content. In particular, we wanted to learn which of the resilience factors are incorporated as part of the program emphasis. We also wanted to learn about how the programs are organized to deliver services, the kinds of barriers they might have faced in implementing the program, and lessons they have learned in addressing those barriers. Finally, we also asked them about how they evaluate their program to determine whether it is successful in promoting resilience. A discussion guide was developed for these semi-structured interviews.

Content of Discussion Guide

The discussion guide was designed to elicit information about program characteristics, program organization, strategies for promoting resilience, barriers to program implementation, and effectiveness evaluation from program representatives. A major objective of these interviews was to identify which of the factors identified through the literature review are central to each program. Thus, we included a list of each of the final factors with a column to check and a space to provide specific examples or comments pertaining to those that are used. Table 3.1 summarizes the interview topic categories

Table 3.1
Program Review Interview Topics and Sample Questions

Topic	Content or Sample Questions
Introduction	Brief project description, oral informed consent
Background information	Individual characteristics (training, position, years with program)
Program organization	How is the program organized? How is the program staffed? What type of training is required of staff?
Strategies for promoting resilience	To what extent are you using/employing the different resilience factors identified by the literature and experts? How does it work? Is this essential for promoting resilience? (Repeat for each factor.)
Other strategies	Is there anything you would like to add to the program? Or eliminate? (Why?)
Barriers to implementation	What are the challenges that you face in running your program?
Effectiveness evaluation	What types of internal evaluation do you conduct on your program? If yes, what do you measure and how do you determine whether it's working? What is the impact for military personnel and their families?
Closing	Thank you. Would you be willing to be contacted again if we have additional questions? Are there any materials that you can share with us (e.g., reports, data, etc.)?

and provides sample content of questions for each category. The full discussion guide is available from the authors on request.

Program Selection and Interview Process

We selected programs to review from among a larger list of 77 programs compiled in consultation with the study sponsor to promote resilience in some way. This longer list is provided in Appendix C. We worked closely with our clients at the DCoE to select a subset of military programs that covered a range of program content (mental, physical, social, and spiritual), that addressed the different audiences (military members, military family, and military leaders), and those that were relatively well developed and/or had potential for being implemented in the military. We also selected a few civilian programs that are not yet adapted to a military setting because they had potential for such application.

Representatives from the 23 programs were contacted using a two-stage process of notification about the study from the DCoE followed by an invitation from RAND to participate. RAND researchers conducted telephone discussions with program staff for up to one hour. Following the interview, the program staff being interviewed received a copy of the notes to ensure that our records were accurate and to add or correct anything in the notes. For some programs we obtained additional documents to supplement the notes. The interview notes were validated by program staff from 13 of the 23 programs.

Data Analysis

Information from the individual program interview notes was transferred to Excel spreadsheets (for program characteristics, resilience factors, barriers, and evaluation). This enabled the research team to view responses to particular topical areas across programs for comparison. The research team reviewed these aggregated spreadsheets and identified key themes in each area.

Findings

Programs and Program Representatives

We obtained information through documents and interviews for 19 of the 20 initially selected programs. We included all three of the components that are now being rolled into the new Comprehensive Soldier Fitness (CSF) program currently being implemented by the Army. The CSF components include

1. the PRP's Master Resilience Trainer program, which is designed to build and field a cadre of Army sergeants who will be certified to teach specific critical thinking skills to their soldiers
2. Battlemind, which is designed to build warriors and leaders with the inner strength to face the realities of the environment with courage and confidence
3. the Assessment of the Army Center for Enhanced Performance (ACEP), which is designed to enhance performance.

CSF features a strategy to increase the overall resilience in the force by enhancing soldiers in the physical, social, spiritual, and family dimensions and is currently undergoing a systematic assessment. We included the Air Force Landing Gear program and the Marine Corps Operational Stress Control and Readiness (OSCAR) programs to represent the different branches of service, as well as the following programs based on study sponsor request: Gallup, Heartmath, Operational Stress Injury Social Support (OSISS), the Corporate Athlete Program, Mindfulness-based Mind Fitness Training (MMFT), and the National Security Agency (NSA) Employee Engagement Program, which is a renamed variant of the Corporate Athlete Program (Loehr and Schwartz, 2001).

The other programs were included to reach a balance across our criteria. For example, we included the Spiritual Warrior Training Program (SWTP) to represent spiritual program content and the Warrior Resilience and Thriving (WRT) program because it is utilized in theater. In addition, during the course of our interviews, we learned that OSISS, a Canadian program, was complemented by preventive efforts at the Joint Speakers Bureau (JSB, which was formerly included in OSISS) so we reviewed both. Similarly, we wanted to include both variants of programs based on the initial Loehr (of the Corporate Athlete Program) and Schwartz partnership, so we added the Energy Project, which is a variant based on Schwartz and McCarthy's energy management concept (Schwartz and McCarthy, 2007). The former is engagement oriented and the latter is energy oriented. These modifications resulted in a review of 23 programs in total (Table 3.2).

It should be noted that a few of the programs we reviewed are not technically programs but were included because they provide information that is relevant for program development. The Marine Resiliency Study is a research project examining trajectories of adaptation to combat over time. In addition, Gallup Consulting has a variety of tools that could be used to develop a program for the military but is not a specific resilience-promoting program in and of itself.

For these 23 programs, we interviewed a total of 43 representatives. In many cases we spoke with a single representative, but in other cases we spoke with more than one person in a group interview (e.g., we spoke to eight program staff for the WRP). Characteristics of these representatives are provided in Table 3.3. Most of the individuals we interviewed were civilians (n=31). In terms of specialty, the majority were trained as clinical psychologists (n=20). Of these 20 psychologists, 16 had doctoral training; among these doctorates, two are child psychologists, one is a sports psychologist, and one is a psychophysiologist. Six had degrees in research psychology. Four were psychia-

Table 3.2
List of Resilience Programs Reviewed

Assessment of the Army Center for Enhanced Performance (ACEP)
Battlemind
Operational Stress Control and Readiness (OSCAR)
Employee Engagement Program (NSA)/Corporate Athlete
Energy Project
Gallup Consulting
HeartMath
Joint Speakers Bureau (JSB)
Landing Gear
Marine Resiliency Study (MRS)
Mindfulness-Based Mind Fitness Training (MMFT)
National Guard Resiliency Program
Operational Stress Injury Social Support (OSISS)
Passport Toward Success
Penn Resiliency Project (PRP)
Preventive Psychological Health Demonstration Project (PPHDP)
Promoting Alternative THinking Strategies (PATHS)
School Mental Health Team (SMHT)
Senior Leader Wellness Enhancement Seminar (SLWES)
Soldier Evaluation for Life Fitness (SELF)
Spiritual Warrior Training Program (SWTP)
Warrior Resiliency Program (WRP)
Warrior Resilience and Thriving (WRT)

Table 3.3
Summary of Program Representative Characteristics

Program Representative Characteristic		Number of Program Representatives
Professional Affiliation		
Military		12
Civilian		31
Educational Background (Degree)		
Psychology	Clinical (Ph.D., Psy.D., or master's degree)	20
	Research (Ph.D.)	6
Medicine	Psychiatry (M.D.)	4
	Nursing (R.N.)	1
Social Work (master's degree)		5
Divinity (M.Div.)		1
Business (M.B.A.)		5
Other or unspecified (Ph.D.)		5

NOTES: Program representatives were categorized as either military or civilian. Some program representatives reported multiple degrees.

trists, and one of the psychiatrists had a specialization in children. Some representatives are physicians ($n=4$), and one is a nurse. We also interviewed five social workers, a chaplain, five people with business degrees, and five from either unspecified or other backgrounds.

Program Characteristics

Below we describe the organizational characteristics of the 23 programs we reviewed. Additional details for each of these programs are provided in brief project descriptions (Appendix D). The brief program descriptions provide the following information:

- Program name
- Hyperlink for website or online documentation
- Concept
- Mission
- Background
- Program content (psychological, physical, social, spiritual)
- Target audience
- Phases of deployment addressed (pre-, during, post-)

- Services provided (characterized by types, locations, delivery modes, intensity, clients served)
- Target audience
- Sponsor/funding

Table 3.4 summarizes some of the program characteristics. Most of the 23 programs emphasize psychological content (e.g., mental, $n=21$ programs). Many of the

Table 3.4
Summary of Program Characteristics

Program Characteristic	Number of Programs (n=23)
Resilience Domain Addressed	
Mental	21
Physical	12
Social	14
Spiritual	8
Target Audience	
Military members	15
Family members	13
Military leaders	8
Adult civilians	5
Children civilians	1
Phases of Military Deployment Addressed	
Predeployment	14
In theater	12
Post-deployment	16
Services	
Workshops or classes	16
Individual meetings	6
Online resources	6
Train the trainer	7
Sponsor/Funding	
DoD	3
Army	8

Table 3.4—Continued

Program Characteristic	Number of Programs (n=23)
Marines/Navy	2
Air Force	1
National Guard	2
Congress	1
Other DoD (NSA)	1
International military (Canadian Forces)	2
University/research institute	4
Private/civilian	7

NOTE: A program may represent more than one domain or audience.

programs also address physical and social content, and fewer address spiritual content ($n=8$). The programs we reviewed spanned the different types of audiences, with most targeting military members and families. Across the programs, all phases of deployment were addressed. The format of services offered were predominantly workshops or classes ($n=16$), with some individual meetings, online information, and training for trainers as well. In terms of sponsorship, we reviewed some DoD programs as well as programs from specific branches of service. We spoke with representatives of one international program (i.e., Canada, with two program arms), one nonmilitary government agency, several private sector programs, and one government agency that provides products and services to DoD, the NSA.

Factors for Promoting Resilience

In this section we review how the 20 factors that promote resilience map to the 23 programs that were reviewed. This information is based on a combination of program documents and interviews. We first provide general findings describing which types of factors are most common across programs, as well as which are least common. We then drill down to the specific factors to highlight unique patterns and provide illustrative examples of each. Figure 3.1 shows the number of programs that incorporate each resilience factor within the levels of the military environment.

General Findings. Among the different programs we reviewed, individual- and unit-level factors were most often targeted by the programs. Five of the seven individual resilience factors were identified as being targets by nearly all of the 23 programs. Most programs incorporate some form of training or education that involves positive thinking ($n=19$), are designed to teach coping skills ($n=17$), train participants for realism ($n=16$), teach behavioral control skills ($n=16$), or teach positive affect ($n=14$). All three of the unit-level factors were incorporated into the programs, with positive

Figure 3.1
Number of Programs Incorporating Resilience Factors (Ordered by Rank)

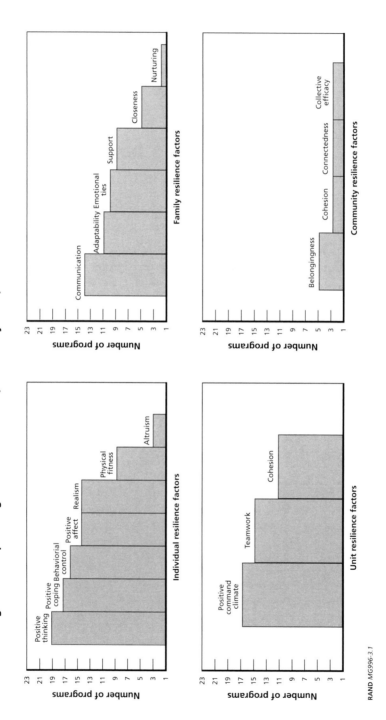

RAND *MG996-3.1*

command climate the most common across programs (*n*=17). In contrast, family factors were somewhat less commonly incorporated into programs designed to promote resilience, in part because fewer of the programs we reviewed were targeted to families. The most common family factor contained in programs was communication (*n*=12). Community-level resilience factors were by far the least common among the programs we reviewed. The most common community-level factor was belongingness (*n*=6). Over half of the programs did not address this level of resilience.

While some programs were comprehensive, incorporating at least half of the 20 factors, others were more targeted. For example, Battlemind addresses 16 different resilience factors. Both the Employee Engagement Program and the Marine Corps COSC (Combat Operational Stress Control) program address 13 factors across the individual, family, and unit levels. Battlemind was reported to have a broad foundation spanning the areas of positive psychology, cognitive restructuring, mindfulness, research on PTSD, unit cohesion, occupational health, organizational leadership, and deployment-related research. One program, the NSA's Employee Engagement Program, reported including all 20 factors in their approach, covering all four levels of resilience in our framework.

In contrast, some programs take a more targeted approach rather than attempting to address all aspects of resilience. For example, the National Guard Resiliency Program focused its curriculum on four factors across individual and unit levels. The Guard's program was rooted in cognitive behavioral therapy, which emphasizes coping and positive thinking as essential individual-level factors. Their program also emphasizes teamwork, describing the process of becoming resilient as a "team journey." One example of a program that concentrates on a particular level is the Passport Toward Success program. Passport targets children and, accordingly, includes more family-level resilience factors. Similarly, the Marine Resiliency Study, which targets active-duty Marines, covers all of the unit-level resilience factors. Figure 3.1 illustrates the prevalence of resilience factors for each type within each level (individual, family, unit, and community).

Findings Specific to Factors. Evidence-informed factors that promote resilience were incorporated into programs in a variety of ways.

Individual-Level Factors.

Positive Coping. Positive coping is incorporated into 18 of the programs we reviewed (see Table 3.5). In the Employee Engagement Program, employees at the NSA walk through different dimensions and talk about areas for improvement. Program staff encourage employees to identify their own coping strategies by raising their consciousness about how they can connect their stress to absences from work. Another example, the JSB, teaches coping skills for military members, their families, and leaders to employ. Service personnel are taught how to deal with the stresses of deployment, families are taught coping skills to help them decompress at home, and leaders are taught how to use practical and easy supportive tools to employ when assisting sub-

Table 3.5
Summary of Resilience Factors Incorporated into Each Program

Resilience Factor	1	2	3	4	5	6	7	8	9	10	11	12	13	14	15	16	17	18	19	20	21	22	23
Individual																							
Positive coping		X	X	X	X			X	X	X	X	X	X	X	X	X	X	X	X	X	X		X
Positive affect	X	X	X	X	X	X	X		X		X			X	X	X	X			X	X		X
Positive thinking	X	X	X	X	X	X	X	X	X		X	X	X	X	X	X	X			X	X	X	X
Realism	X	X	X	X	X	X		X	X		X			X	X	X	X			X	X	X	X
Behavioral control	X	X		X	X	X	X	X	X		X		X	X	X	X	X	X		X			X
Physical fitness		X	X	X	X			X	X			X				X				X			
Altruism				X	X	X																	
Family																							
Emotional ties		X	X	X	X			X	X				X	X	X			X					
Communication		X	X	X	X	X		X			X		X	X	X		X	X	X				X
Support		X	X	X	X			X	X				X	X	X								
Closeness		X	X	X	X									X									
Nurturing						X								X									
Adaptability	X	X	X		X		X	X	X	X	X		X	X	X								
Unit																							
Positive command climate	X	X	X	X	X	X	X	X	X	X	X	X	X	X	X	X				X	X	X	X
Teamwork	X	X	X	X	X	X	X	X	X	X	X	X		X	X	X				X	X		X
Cohesion	X	X	X		X		X	X	X	X	X			X	X	X				X	X		X

Table 3.5—Continued

Resilience Factor	1	2	3	4	5	6	7	8	9	10	11	12	13	14	15	16	17	18	19	20	21	22	23
Community																							
Belongingness	X				X	X	X										X				X		X
Cohesion					X		X												X				
Connectedness					X		X													X			
Collective efficacy	X				X		X																

NOTE: 1 = Assessment of the Army Center for Enhanced Performance (ACEP). 2 = Battlemind. 3 = Operational Stress Control and Readiness. 4 = Employee Engagement Program (NSA)/Corporate Athlete. 5 = Energy Project. 6 = Gallup Consulting. 7 = HeartMath. 8 = Joint Speakers Bureau. 9 = Landing Gear. 10 = Marine Resilience Study (MRS). 11= Mindfulness-Based Mind Fitness Training (MMFT). 12 = National Guard Resiliency Program. 13 = Operational Stress Injury Social Support (OSISS). 14 = Passport Toward Success. 15 = Penn Resiliency Project (PRP). 16 = Preventive Psychological Health Demonstration Project (PPHDP). 17 = Promoting Alternative THinking Strategies (PATHS). 18 = School Mental Health Team (SMHT). 19 = Senior Leader Wellness Enhancement Seminar (SLWES). 20 = Soldier Evaluation for Life Fitness (SELF). 21 = Spiritual Warrior Training Program (SWTP). 22 = Warrior Resiliency Program (WRP). 23 = Warrior Resilience and Thriving (WRT) ordinates with prevention and early intervention. The MMFT program encourages the use of coping to foster a move from avoidant-style coping mechanisms (ignoring, denying, suppressing, distracting) toward active coping mechanisms, such as acceptance of stressors and decentered relationship to stressors. They indicate that doing so creates space and builds the capacity to work creatively with the problem at hand.

Positive Affect. Fifteen of the programs reviewed incorporate positive affect as a factor to promote resilience. The PRP, in particular, is a pioneer in the field, with a well-established curriculum based on positive psychology that makes positive affect a central factor by training soldiers about positive emotions and promoting optimism. HeartMath teaches individuals how to implement techniques focused on positive emotions to reduce stress and negative affect along with biofeedback. Their Shift and Reset tool does this by draining negative mental and emotional reactions and activating a positive state before addressing stressors. SELF employs positive affect by incorporating humor into provider interviews, as appropriate, and is also discussed in the context of soldiers' posttraumatic growth inventory results. Another example is Passport Toward Success, a reunion support program designed to help children and families reconnect after a military deployment. It comprises activities to help military children and youth learn and practice skills that will help them with reintegration and also help them to reconnect with parents following separation. A fundamental aim of the program is to increase positive affect through increased awareness of emotional needs among family members.

Positive Thinking. Positive thinking techniques are evident in 20 of the programs reviewed. For example, the ACEP program employs a variety of positive thinking tools—including goal-setting, mental skills foundations/concentration, and integrating imagery—to help soldiers and family members achieve the mental strength necessary to reach their potential throughout their entire lives. The program is specifically designed to facilitate optimal human performance while promoting and contributing to overall hardiness and resiliency. The PRP program includes a range of cognitive behavioral techniques from the field of positive psychology. Three of the eight days of the program are focused on teaching soldiers to avoid thinking traps and challenge negative beliefs. The WRT program emphasizes rationality and critical thinking by teaching soldiers how to recognize, dispute, and replace irrational beliefs that lead to emotional suffering, poor performance, and combat operational stress. The WRT also teaches rational emotive behavior therapy (REBT). REBT is taught at the unit level to soldiers, medics, peer coaches, and leaders and is practiced in the Army Medical department course for mental health technicians. The PATHS program also stresses positive thinking techniques by training teachers through interactive lessons to choose effective conflict-resolution strategies.

Realism. Realism is a feature of 15 programs that we reviewed. Some of the ways in which realism is used include training to foster internal locus of control. For example, MMFT helps participants gain a sense of self-efficacy through an increased ability to regulate and tolerate the activation of the autonomic nervous system in response to stress, as well as an increased ability to tolerate and modulate unpleasant emotional states. By learning how to use focused attention to re-regulate the body and mind following stress, they learn to accept what is beyond their control and cannot be changed. Landing Gear teaches as a core competency to "accept that change is a part of living; move toward your goals," and Marine COSC attempts to restore self-confidence and self-esteem as part of its mitigation function. The PATHS program trains teachers of elementary-aged children to enhance mastery by increasing social competency and emotional control. Teaching self-regulation and self-awareness is also a core focus of the PRP.

Behavioral Control Skills. Behavioral control skills are taught as part of 17 programs, including HeartMath, which focuses on self-regulation. HeartMath's resilience programs for military personnel are based on first identifying the psychophysiological state of coherence (resonance) as an optimal state of emotional, cognitive, and physical functioning. Coherence allows individuals to build, maintain, and sustain resilience. Coherence-building is accomplished using a biofeedback technology program that was developed out of the basic research. One of the fundamental goals of the Air Force's Landing Gear program is to encourage airmen to look for opportunities for self-discovery. MMFT teaches improved emotional intelligence (knowing one's own emotions, regulating one's emotions, recognizing emotions in others, handing relationships effectively). Improved emotion regulation can lead to increased tolerance for challenging and adverse situations and people, and it also leads to less likelihood of impulsive, reactive, or inappropriate behavior.

Physical Fitness. Nine programs involve some element of physical fitness. For example, in addition to emphasizing many of the psychological principles, Battlemind also emphasizes the importance of getting plenty of sleep for maintaining resilience. Landing Gear staff plan to develop additional training modules that teach airmen to take care of themselves by exercising and getting adequate sleep and nutrition. For the NSA's Employee Engagement Program, the concept of energy is an integral component of the training. This area, covering fitness and nutrition, is addressed in the physical dimension of their training. The PPHDP is testing three different levels of resilience interventions: organizational, individual, and embedded/unit level. In addition to other resilience factors, the program teaches heart rhythm coherence, cardiorespiratory function, and blood pressure control.

Altruism. Altruism is addressed by three of the programs that we reviewed. The Energy Project addresses altruism through a spiritual training module. The Gallup Consulting program's Clifton StrengthsFinder and Well-Being Finder tools provide a strategy for promoting resilience in military leadership and personnel. These tools increase awareness of strengths, which leads to higher self-awareness and self-efficacy and ultimately to increased altruism.

Family-Level Factors.

Emotional Ties. Turning to factors that promote resilience at the family level, we found ten programs that incorporate the concept of emotional ties into their approaches. For example, Battlemind emphasizes the importance of soldiers' relationships back home as a source of support and strength. JSB includes family education about what to expect when a military member is deployed. Skills are taught for how to cope with situations that occur while the family is separated. The SMHT program provides a wide range of preventive programs that facilitate adaptive adjustment to stressors for military youth by providing a "socio-emotional culture" within the school and the family. Deployment groups, parenting groups, and acculturation groups all strive to build interpersonal connections among parents and between parents and schools.

Family Communication. Family communication is a factor that is incorporated into 14 programs we reviewed. The COSC program aims to strengthen Marines using a broad array of techniques, including communication. The goal is to build communication into the culture by putting all positive leadership duties (e.g., building trust) into a psychological framework. OSISS employs communication by encouraging military members to express their feelings to loved ones. The Indiana National Guard, through the Passport Toward Success program, specifically addresses connection and communication within families by increasing the ability for children and families to understand the benefits of appropriate communication following deployment. SLWES also implicitly incorporates communication through breakout discussions about stress and how it is dealt with between leaders and their families (spouses and children).

Family Support. Family support is a feature of nine programs. For example, OSISS offers social support by peer support coordinators and also by OSISS volunteers known as peer support helpers, who are persons suffering from the consequences of an operational stress injury (OSI) or other injuries related to service. A few programs addressed family support indirectly, in that they do not necessarily train or educate family members but do include family-based content. For example, the Employee Engagement Program at NSA includes individual action plans for change, many of which have been focused on improving family relationships. The Energy Project also addresses the importance of partner support to help employees change behaviors and increase capacity for performing under pressure, but family members are not directly involved.

Family Closeness. Family closeness was a concept central to five of the programs reviewed. Battlemind emphasizes closeness in terms of family bonds. The training provides modules for military spouses that use a developmental approach to mental health skill building timed to the specific phases of the soldiers' career and deployment cycle. The COSC program incorporates closeness through their program within its strengthen function. That program component includes training activities that emphasize love and intimacy for families. Passport Toward Success focuses on activities for children and their parents, in conjunction with seamless transition activities to enhance closeness through fostering trust in others and increasing awareness of emotional needs.

Family Nurturing. Family nurturing (parenting skills) was a factor present for only two programs we reviewed. Gallup Consulting representatives reported that their programs equip parents with the knowledge and tools that will enable them to build on their parenting skills and develop an increased capacity to nurture their children. They inform their participants that building a "strength-based culture" at home promotes a more nurturing and positive environment. Passport Toward Success teaches resiliency skills through family connection exercises, which help military youth better cope with parental separation as a result of military deployment.

Family Adaptability. Ten programs incorporate the concept of family adaptability in some manner. Battlemind teaches skills that families learn during deployment to help them cope with separation of loved ones. For example, a key message in Battlemind is that "families must be able to function effectively without you" and there are skills that families can learn during deployment to make them better able to manage during deployment. A central message incorporated into the Landing Gear training is that family adaptability means that one must learn to accept that some circumstances cannot be changed. The JSB provides family education about what to expect when the military member is deployed and encourages families to be flexible. Practical skills are taught, including how to cope with role changes while the family is separated. This component is based on a program developed by the U.S. Naval Special Warfare Center, which is rooted in sports performance psychology and applies goal-setting techniques to help families adapt to military life.

Unit-Level Factors. Unit-level factors associated with resilience are particularly important for the military context and relatively prevalent across the different programs that we reviewed.

Positive Command Climate. Positive command climate is a factor incorporated into materials for nearly all of the programs (n=18 of 23) we reviewed. As an example, MMFT teaches leaders to become better at recognizing emotions in themselves and others and to become more open to feedback from subordinates. In a pilot study, leaders reported that they gained capacity with prioritizing tasks for themselves and for the unit in general. The SELF program is another example in which commanders are trained to provide suggestions for improving unit cohesion and leadership effectiveness, where needed. SWTP tasks chaplains with finding "hot spots" in a company and then providing spiritual support that helps the service member and command.

Teamwork. Teamwork is a critical feature of military life and was identified as a component of 16 of the programs reviewed. The National Guard Resilience Program materials emphasize that "learning to be resilient is a team journey." COSC, which includes the Marine Operational Stress Control and Readiness (OSCAR) embedded mental health providers, has teamwork at its core. For example, the OSCAR component requires mental health providers, corpsmen, and Marine noncommissioned officers to spend as much time as possible with battalions and companies in their regiment, as far forward as is feasible, to provide prevention, early identification, and effective treatment at the lowest level possible. Team members work together to provide (1) command consultation, (2) outreach (presence in the field), (3) surveillance-identification-monitoring, (4) resilience promotion training and mentoring, (5) liaison with other sources of support and care, (6) intervention (advanced stress first aid, unit level interventions, individual treatment), and (7) caregiver support. Commanders also play a role that includes (1) welcoming OSCAR personnel into units and staffs, (2) learning OSCAR team capabilities and limitations, (3) training OSCAR personnel in unit's mission, capabilities, and culture, (4) giving clear guidance, (5) providing feedback, and (6) submitting lessons learned regarding OSCAR. OSCAR is teaching leaders COSC as a resilience component. The aim is to have intensive implementation in the infantry and a clinical presence there to enable more clinical intervention. These teams are organic and fully integrated into the units. They have clearly defined roles in both training and operational environments. They must be present in the field during training and operations, at least at the company level. They must be visible and become known and trusted by unit members with line commander ownership in units. The primary focus is to improve psychological health of the unit as a whole. A secondary focus is to identify and treat individuals with mental health problems, using a multidisciplinary team approach.

Unit Cohesion. Unit cohesion is also essential to the military mission and is present in materials for 12 programs we reviewed. A major component of Battlemind is the concept of a "battle buddy." Soldiers are encouraged to talk to each other to identify potential sources of stress. This approach prepares soldiers and leaders mentally for the rigors of combat and other military deployments, assists soldiers in their successful transition back home, prepares soldiers with the skills to assist their battle buddy during deployment as well as to transition back home, and prepares soldiers to possibly deploy again in support of all types of military operations, including additional combat tours. The rationale behind SWTP is that the morale of a unit is related to the spiritual well-being of the individual. Spiritual health focuses on nonmaterial parts of humanity, such as emotions, will, thoughts, faith, and purpose in life. A healthy spiritual life produces healthy behaviors, which directly affect the quality and readiness of the individual and unit in the areas of cohesion, inspired leadership, team building, unity, and collaboration. The SELF materials for commanders contain suggestions for improving unit cohesion and leadership effectiveness.

Community-Level Factors.

Belongingness. While less prevalent, belongingness was discussed as a part of seven programs. The Gallup Consulting program provides a good example. One of the program's tools is the Well-Being Index (WBI) and World Poll. The WBI assesses overall well-being, which includes levels of belongingness in a civic environment, such as a military base or an outside community. Military leadership and decisionmakers can subsequently use this information from the survey to measure overall levels of belong-ingness. The WBI can serve as a benchmark across bases and communities with large populations across the country. This information can be used to guide program and policy decisions to improve health and well-being for military personnel, their families, and their respective communities. SMHTs use belongingness to promote resilience by arranging formal linkages with community agencies, as well as building interpersonal connections among parents and between parents and schools.

Community Cohesion. Only three programs incorporate community cohesion as a concept in how they enhance resilience. These include the Energy Project, which uses an Organizational Energy Audit (OEA) that identifies and quantifies the way that an organization's current practices (policies, procedures, rules, and reward/recognition systems) and culture (explicit and implicit values, beliefs, norms, and expectations) influence people's capacity to perform at their best. The OEA includes a comprehensive site visit to assess how the organizational environment influences the energy and engagement of employees, one-on-one interviews, focus groups with key leaders and stakeholders, and an online survey of a statistically valid sample of all employees. An OEA report serves as a roadmap by which organizations can identify the areas in which specific policies, practices, or implicit cultural messages are influencing people's energy. Following the OEA, the program typically consults with a designated team of senior leaders to help them design, implement, and execute new organizational initiatives that enable employees to more efficiently manage their own energy. HeartMath also engages in a community cohesion effort. They connect with veteran service agencies within local communities (American Veterans, Vietnam Veterans, etc.) to establish partnerships that will help deliver programs to the military families at the community level. HeartMath is also trying to leverage elements of community resilience—not just address them—through a collaborative program to take training to the communities. The goal is to establish family groups during predeployment so that the groups can communicate with the military on issues related to the deployed individual or group of individuals. These family groups can take care of individual families while the service member is deployed. In this way, they build resilience in that particular community rather than having a broader regional focus. The goal is to shift the focus from bases or units to communities to promote resilience in the military. Community cohesion is also a part of the SWTP program, to the extent that it is enhanced through intentional ministry within the unit.

Community Connectedness. Community connectedness was also identified as a resilience factor present in three programs. A key component of the Energy Project process is to increase people's awareness of the costs and benefits of their current behaviors. At the same time, they are committed to moving people from intellectual understanding to enduring behavioral change. To that end, they teach participants to build "positive rituals"—highly specific energy-management strategies that become automatic over time. Building rituals is the ultimate payoff in their work and ensures that participants return to their jobs not just with ideas about how to change, but with a step-by-step process for doing so. This process strengthens individual employees' connections with their employer organization, which enhances performance and ultimately leads employers to build clear competitive advantage and fuel more-enduring high performance by systematically meeting the multidimensional needs of their employees. As part of the effort to engage veterans in the community (described above), HeartMath is also enhancing the quality and number of connections that people have in their community. Specifically, they are enhancing communication, teamwork, and goal clarity through these connections. Again, SWTP helps a healthy spiritual life to produce healthy behaviors, which in turn are related to resilience. This is done, in part, with group events within the military community connecting soldiers, veterans, and family.

Collective Efficacy. The last factor, collective efficacy, is a component discussed in three of the 23 programs. These include Battlemind, which incorporates the Soldier's Creed into its materials and through their tools reemphasizes the importance of being part of something larger than oneself. The Energy Project also reported incorporating the idea of collective efficacy, to the extent that enhanced individual performance leads to strengthened ability for employees to work together productively. Finally, the HeartMath program includes a resource called Power Tools for Inner Quality, which trains on creating a caring culture and increasing job satisfaction. It teaches participants to use emotional restructuring—the Heart Lock-In technique—to reduce stress and increase physiological coherence. Specifically, the approach includes teaching participants to "appreciate" by taking time out to notice and be grateful for the positive aspects of one's life, and "neutralize" distressing emotions.

To summarize, three of the programs incorporated all five of the resilience factors that had the most support based on the literature review (positive coping, positive affect, positive thinking, family support, and belongingness). Six of the programs incorporated the five factors with the strongest evidence across the individual and family levels of resilience. Generally speaking, all of the programs reviewed in this monograph include at least one of the resilience factors that is strongly supported, mostly at the individual level. Of the seven programs that address broader community-level factors, which are less well-researched and therefore have less evidence in the literature, all include belongingness along with the three strongest individual-level evidence-informed resilience factors.

Barriers to Program Implementation

Program representatives were asked to describe challenges they faced in implementing and operating their programs and to reflect on any lessons learned that would be helpful to others interested in implementing similar resilience-based programs. We found that although there were some barriers specific to each program, consistent themes emerged across programs. In addition, general barriers to program implementation and sustainment were more commonly reported and emphasized as more important than challenges specific to resilience content. Programs also shared strategies they found successful in navigating these barriers. A summary of common barriers faced across programs appears in Table 3.6.

Lack of Leadership Support. The most commonly cited barrier to program implementation was related to challenges gaining or maintaining buy-in from military commanders. As one program official stated, "There is a strong need for leadership support. There is tension in some places where leadership is thought of as a coercive element. Noncoercive endorsement is key." Program representatives who reported success in implementation also cited positive command climate as the most important factor contributing to program success. One program representative described how an effective resilience program was terminated after a change in command because the new leader was less supportive of the program.

According to the program representatives we spoke with, leaders also influence how the program is integrated into existing training efforts, which can influence the success of implementation. One program representative described this example: "To make any resilience training effective, leadership has to value the training as providing a foundational, general-purpose skill that is worthy of time on the training schedule.

Table 3.6
Summary of Reported Barriers to Program Implementation

Barrier	Number of Programs Addressing Barrier	Examples
Lack of leadership support	13	"Supportive leadership . . . can model change in their own behavior and also serve as a 'strong internal champion' for the program." "When communication from the top down is not as clear, families may not get relevant information or feel particularly encouraged to attend. There is higher participation when commanders' families participate in the program."
Problems with logistics	12	"Identifying appropriate periods of measurement within the military is an ongoing challenge." "There are many demands on training time . . . sometimes training time is cut short in order to continue the mission."
Limited funding to sustain program	8	"The business process [of] traditional systems works against efforts to provide a prevention oriented system. Currently, they are tied to a system that rewards for patient encounters." "We started with some seed money to develop the program and got additional support from local representatives. It will be important to get ongoing support to further develop and expand the program."
Poor fit within the military	8	"It is a challenge to figure out how to present the material in an effective way, e.g., self-care and self regulation can be presented as part of self-sustainment."
Mental health stigma	5	"Soldier's reaction is 'Why do we need this touchy-feely course?' It is sometimes hard to get through to senior leadership the importance of addressing these issues prior to deployment."

In one instance, a detachment commander found [our program] and asked to be in [a study we were conducting]—however, the commander three levels above did not believe the training was a good use of time. The outcome was that we had to arrange our training schedule to be adjacent to the existing training schedule. As a result, the trainees felt that the program was not fully integrated into the schedule and took away from their free time. The program had the feel of being added on as an extra or an afterthought when it should have been a priority."

Leadership was also viewed as important in breaking down negative attitudes associated with program participation. When commanders participate in the program, are physically present, or otherwise demonstrate they value and use the program themselves, participants are more willing to attend, and this facilitates implementation. As one program observed, "Particularly for mandatory programs, strong direction and support (both conceptual and visible) from the commander promotes participant interest and motivation. Preferably, the commander (not program staff) will present the value of the program to participants and will maintain coordinated efforts with program staff. The best scenario is when this type of training is emphasized as just as important as other aspects of training."

Strategies that program representatives used to overcome less positive command climate included early investment in communicating often with leadership, emphasizing the potential for positive military outcomes, and sharing preliminary outcome data. One program utilized the familiar military framework of leadership enhancement and building the warrior ethos to introduce their resilience program—they explained how their program supported Army values. Another program provided a detailed strategy for gaining command support in their implementation guide, which included giving measurable outcomes and showing how participation would benefit the commander's management of the unit.

Problems with Logistics. Training program staff, maintaining adequate numbers of staff, acquiring adequate physical space, establishing methods of quality assurance, and coordinating program activities to avoid duplication were among many cited logistical barriers to implementation. Many programs began as small pilot efforts, and expansion to broader audiences was often limited by the program's ability to "scale up." A related logistical issue of concern was how best to conduct follow-up assessments for programs that tracked outcomes. As one program mentioned, "It is difficult to get people to come back and retake all of the assessment. The return rate ranges from 23 percent to 68 percent." Other programs struggled with determining which outcomes to measure. Many program representatives felt that implementation of programs within the military required additional approvals that impeded progress. However, one program that worked with schools faced similar challenges and established "memorandums of understanding" across groups to formalize approval prior to implementation. Regarding physical space, some programs felt that they sacrificed efficacy in order to benefit from the convenience of conducting the program on base: "We learned that having break-out areas that were small enough so that people felt comfortable that whatever they were saying was private was very important, and that more flexible times for seminars were needed. We conducted the sessions on the base, but we now think that a hotel with many breakout rooms would be a better location."

Limited Funding to Sustain Program. Many programs noted the challenge of obtaining and maintaining a funding stream to sustain their resilience programs. Many programs started with seed money and struggled to identify sources of sustainable funding. Funding sources varied from program to program, but a funding barrier potentially unique to resilience programs is the lack of alignment with existing traditional mental health care or general training funding streams. Many programs could be characterized as preventive in nature in terms of mental health outcomes and are structured to function as a general military training program with a novel focus on promoting optimal psychological performance. This can create a challenge when competing for funding across different streams that have different priorities and outcomes of interest. As one program commented, "The DoD budget requires health care funds to be spent within a narrow definition of health care [delivery] that does not always support ideas that may build resilience. Funding may have to come from a different pot of money." Other programs found resources within the state or training budget to support their efforts. Although programs had few suggestions of how to overcome this structural barrier (e.g., that resilience programs are prevention-oriented and not housed within traditional health care), some were hopeful that a growing awareness of and interest in building resilience within the military would eventually translate into more easily accessible sources of program funding.

Difficulty Aligning Barriers Specific to Resilience Factor Content Within the Military. A few program representatives cited issues related to program content or the structure of the program as important barriers. Related to the choice of topics, one program noted, "Stress as a topic got quickly worn out. There was also a need to make sure that participants gain concrete takeaway skills. Structured topics worked better, as well as focusing on specific subtopics (not just general stress, but how your children are coping, how has this affected your communication)." One program representative noted that "Interventions like [teaching] cognitive behavioral [skills] may not be as effective predeployment because soldiers are in such a cognitively depleted state . . . with high levels of anxiety and depression: soldiers are anticipating separation, being in harm's way; there is renegotiation of the family structure; training days are extremely long—13 to 16 hours seven days a week. There is a lot of stopping and starting—soldiers are trying to fit in all sorts of different certifications—and then trying to solidify certain skills sets at the same time. The key is to have enough lead time with the training so that trainees can be practicing over a period of time before deployment." The challenge for soldiers is to practice and solidify these new skills when they are preparing for deployments with long training days, as opposed to approaching resilience programs as a one-time "stand-down." According to one program representative, "The problem is that the training gets watered down into a script instead of really being absorbed."

Program representatives also discussed the need for modification and updating of program content to ensure (1) engagement and (2) appropriateness. As one representative noted "A major lesson learned from the cyclical aspects of the training is how to address overexposure. This issue was less relevant to one-time programs. Refreshing the training on a regular basis to keep the deployment-cycle training relevant and interesting to soldiers is crucial in the setting of multiple deployments to prevent the perception that this is a low-priority training. Also, providing a refresher course for soldier support training helps renew their skills and get feedback." Another representative also noted that "Programs that target families need to develop age-appropriate program content."

A related program administration barrier cited by one program involved the use of civilian personnel. When civilian programs are adapted to the military, key program staff may need to overcome a lack of familiarity with the military. The program developed close partnerships with military personnel and utilized workgroups to address this issue.

These content and structural administration barriers were thought to negatively affect program effectiveness and acceptability. According to program representatives, adopting a flexible content approach early in the development process was important for some programs to ensure an adequate fit for the military population. Programs that had a more structured implementation process also faced challenges; program representatives noted that they needed to invest more resources in ensuring the fidelity of trainers or use certified trainers, which may have created additional burden to participate.

Mental Health Stigma. Distinguishing resilience programs from traditional mental health programs can be important to facilitate engagement with service members and reduce stigma. Many programs we reviewed were designed for nonclinical groups or for the general military population and their families. Program representatives often spoke of their programs as preventive but noted that the programs were often perceived as treatment or clinical entities by service members. Other resilience programs were embedded within traditional mental health treatment systems, which complicated efforts to reduce stigma and normalize participation. As one program representative commented, "One of our greatest barriers to messaging was soldiers' previous negative association with behavioral health—they were imagining they were going to get more of the same—preconception of dread . . . or the message that they are doomed to get PTSD." To address this barrier, program representatives reported investing considerable effort emphasizing the strength-building aspects of their services, and many utilized a comparison with physical fitness training to relate the nature and goals of their program. Other program representatives indicated that they simply highlighted the preventive aspects of their program to encourage participation.

Summary of Barriers. In summary, the most common and critical barrier to program success (as reported by program representatives) was lack of support from military leadership. Other reported barriers included logistical challenges related to coordinating training efforts and program events in the context of a dynamic and demanding military environment. Funding was also mentioned as a barrier to sustainment and expansion of many resilience programs; the specific issues of funding were related to bridging mental health care and military training paradigms—neither of which are fully aligned with resilience paradigms. Despite a range of barriers that were endorsed, many programs were able to overcome them and shared their lessons learned and strategies for success.

Evaluation of Program Effectiveness

This section highlights findings from the program review associated with how programs evaluate their own effectiveness. We summarize basic themes generated from the notes taken during personal interviews rather than from detailed examination of published results or program materials. This approach limited our ability to compare programs. For example, if the notes about a program do not mention using satisfaction ratings for program planning, one cannot infer that the program did not evaluate their program in that manner. Thus, we do not compare programs across characteristics, such as outcomes measured, but instead provide general themes, with selected examples of programs that are representative of the themes. In addition, all programs reviewed contained multiple factors that have been shown to be associated with resilience. Evidence of the effectiveness of the overall program itself does not isolate which of the multiple factors contributed most to good outcomes.

Few Programs Have Formally Evaluated Their Effectiveness

- Of the resilience programs/studies reviewed, relatively few had conducted and published RCTs or quasi-experimental studies to show that their programs result in better outcomes. Further, when more rigorous scientific evidence is available to demonstrate the impact of the program, much of the evidence is based on studies of the program's use in nonmilitary populations.
- No formal evaluations have been conducted to date by Landing Gear, the War-Fighter Diaries component of the National Guard Resiliency Program, OSCAR (although an evaluation is under way), the Senior Leader Wellness Enhancement Seminar (SLWES), SELF, WRT, or U Penn on Master Resilience Training. Some of these programs have requested formal evaluation, but they need additional support and funding in order for evaluations to be undertaken. Almost all of those interviewed saw the need for longitudinal studies of the effectiveness of their programs.

Peer-reviewed evidence on program effectiveness in military populations comes primarily through studies of Battlemind, while other studies of military populations have not yet been published.

- The Battlemind program has conducted 5–6 randomized controlled trials of different aspects of the program (see Adler et al., 2009a, and Adler et al., 2009b, for example). In addition, they are planning a full RCT for 2011 of the Battlemind program for basic combat training. Post-deployment Battlemind training has been adapted by the British military and is being evaluated in a group RCT.
- The ACEP program has a research arm charged with assessing the efficacy of their program in order to develop evidence-based future program capabilities. ACEP staff are currently overseeing 12 studies. Approximately seven scientific manuscripts have been generated, but as of the interview date, none had yet been published. Currently, the ACEP program is assessing the efficacy of their program in the initial entry training environment and conducting an RCT at Fort Jackson. The group RCT comparing eight hours of ACEP education with eight hours of military history education was recently completed. The trial was delivered across eight weeks of basic combat training in 20–40 minute sessions in 47 platoons (23 ACEP and 24 military history). Preliminary data (received from LTC Burbelo) show equivalent ratings of satisfaction and relevance, but soldiers who received ACEP education fared better than soldiers who received military history education on some performance indicators, such as marksmanship and physical fitness, and also used more mental fitness skills (self-talk, relaxation, imagery, and self-confidence). ACEP trainees also reported less use of negative thinking and worrying. In addition, the ACEP program has several other studies in progress focused on warrior transition units, family readiness groups, rifle marksmanship and combat performance, and language school performance. The recent ACEP review of the literature on applied mental skills training interventions (personal communication, LTC Burbelo) noted a lack of research in military populations for several key components of the ACEP model (e.g., self-confidence, self-talk, goal setting, imagery). Since building self-confidence is one of the key components of the ACEP model, ACEP investigators suggest that more research needs to be conducted to explore interventions for improving this mental skill within military populations. Similarly, goal setting, which enhances motivation, may be a valuable topic for future research with military populations.
- The HeartMath program has conducted some controlled research studies, as yet unpublished, including an evaluation of Kansas National Guard returning soldiers with PTSD and an evaluation of a preventive model utilizing phone-based health coaching.

Several studies related to resilience in military populations are in the planning stages or have just been funded, so as yet no data are available from them.

- The Marine Resiliency Study is enrolling 2,300–2,400 members of the 1st Marine Division in a prospective study to gather information on the various trajectories of adaptation to combat. They have completed a pilot study to test the feasibility of the larger study and have started enrolling members for the main study. Data will be gathered within the month prior to deployment, one week after deployment, and three and six months after deployment.
- The MMFT program has also completed a pilot study and is in the process of planning a large study to test the efficacy of different components of their program in a predeployment context. Their study will be an RCT comparing a control group to versions of MMFT that are different lengths.
- The PPHDP has recently been funded and will be conducting a program evaluation of community and health outcomes in six Army installations. Comparison data will be collected from a matched cohort and compared with the intervention groups in order to determine whether this health intervention designed to build resiliency should be added to existing DoD health care programs.
- The WRP, which is a collection of programs and initiatives that are being developed over time, has a research division that will conduct needs assessment, program evaluation, and process improvement studies. In particular, they plan to conduct outcome studies on the effectiveness of provider resiliency training programs and other training programs within WRP.
- The Master Resilience Training program conducted by the PRP is a component of comprehensive soldier fitness and will be evaluated using the Global Assessment Tool (GAT), which soldiers will complete every two years throughout their career. The soldiers will be able to monitor their own growth using the tool, and the Army will analyze the aggregate data. In addition, the Army is planning a more rigorous and independent controlled trial.

Much of the evidence on program effectiveness comes from studies based on nonmilitary populations. These studies focus on different client populations, and the programs themselves are modified for each client. This makes evaluation of one program, such as the Energy Project or Gallup project, difficult.

- The Energy Project grew out of working with elite performers in a variety of fields. They tailor their programs to meet client delivery needs and are flexible in regards to what works logistically and/or culturally within a particular organization.
- Gallup has designed hundreds of measurement-based consulting engagements and conducted different types of analyses at both the individual and organi-

zational level. Numerous publications and books are available on the different Gallup tools, and results are specific to different clients.

- Components of the HeartMath program are research-based positive emotion–focused approaches, which are based on two decades of research and field studies conducted by the Institute of HeartMath. RCTs and other quasi-experimental designs have been conducted in multiple settings.
- The PRP is backed by 19 controlled studies with more than 2,000 children and adolescents. Their program, which is based on evidence-based treatment for depression and anxiety, has been modified and tailored for use in the Army's Master Resilience Training Project.
- The PATHS study has conducted four clinical trials over the past 15 years, several observational studies, and one RCT.

Many Different Types of Outcomes Have Been Gathered to Track Program Effectiveness by the Programs Themselves

Most programs gathered feedback either through satisfaction ratings or qualitative interviews to establish program feasibility or to refine and improve the program.

- SLWES, SELF, the Energy Project, HeartMath, and the Flashforward project of the National Guard Resiliency Program all use ratings or interviews for program improvement. Others use post-class/training feedback surveys (Employee Engagement Program/Corporate Athlete, the Energy Project, JSB, OSISS, Passport Toward Success, WRT) and in some cases follow subjects over time (e.g., Employee Engagement Program/Corporate Athlete).
- The SMHT/Army School-Based Project tracks clinical effort and impact on participants during and at the end of treatment.
- SWTP gathers information about service members during several phases of training in order to identify soldiers in need of attention and to provide feedback to commanders.
- Finally, some programs collect information about emotional and behavioral health–related needs (such as evidence of antisocial behavior or brief validated measures of depression, anxiety, anger, relationship quality, unit cohesion, suicidality, or alcohol and substance use) in order to connect service members to professionals who can help if needed (e.g., OSISS, SELF, SWTP).

When clinical data are gathered, frequently included are measures of mental health symptoms, often including measures of depression, PTSD, anxiety, and general distress.

These outcomes have been used in some cases to monitor the effectiveness of the program and in other cases to determine need for psychiatric care or further assessment. Other mental health–related outcomes that were measured among program participants included aggressive behavior, anger, positive affect, self-regulation, mind-fulness, attention, memory, mood states, sleep problems, suicidality, cognitive perfor-mance, and, for children, reduced problem behaviors.

The type of outcome measure gathered depends on the goals of the study, target population, and resources available for evaluation efforts.

- The Employee Engagement Program, which includes creating an energy profile as part of participation, gathers information from participants on biometrics (e.g., cholesterol, blood sugar, body fat analysis, body mass index [BMI]), fitness, and weight management, among others.
- HeartMath focuses on the physiological effects of positive emotions and uses an emWave tool to measure heart rate variability over time. However, a variety of other outcomes are also measured, depending on the type of study. For example, in education studies they evaluate test anxiety, risky behaviors, improved test scores, classroom behavior, and academic performance. In the workplace they assess productivity, goal clarity, and job satisfaction. In addition, HeartMath has developed a Personal and Organizational Quality Assessment Tool (POQA) and their own stress and well-being surveys.
- The MMFT study, which focuses on building resilience through mindfulness training, will be evaluating their program with neurocognitive testing of atten-tion and memory using electroencephalography (EEG) recordings of brain-wave activity during cognitive behavioral tasks. The study will also include self-reported measures of stress and resilience and cortisol profiling to measure the body's phys-iological stress response. Their pilot study measured cognitive capabilities using the Profile of Mood States, the Perceived Stress Scale, the Five-Facet Mindfulness Questionnaire, the Positive and Negative Affect Scale, and the Personal Outlook Scale, among others.

Outcomes tended to be measured most frequently at the individual level, with fewer assessments mentioned at the family and organizational level (includ-ing unit).

- The Energy Program, which has not been conducted in the military to date, includes metrics that vary depending on the client organization. Individual com-panies focus on measures of productivity, engagement, and work satisfaction.
- Gallup has specific tools (such as the Clifton StrengthsFinder, the Well-Being Finder, and the Q-12/Hope tools) that they use at the individual level to monitor behavioral change, such as higher levels of engagement at work and in life (i.e., they track program outcomes, such as well-being, engagement, health, self-efficacy, hope, and altruism). They have a StrengthsExplorer tool for children ages 14–17 and a StrengthQuest tool for college-age students. However, Gallup also focuses

at the organizational level on overall work unit engagement results, scorecards, benchmarks, performance impact measures, and other client-requested outcomes.

- The Passport Toward Success program focuses on the family. Their targeted outcomes include improved sense of connection among family members, increased understanding about the benefits of appropriate communication, increased use of coping skills among family members, and increased awareness of emotional needs. To gather this information, they collect data from children who are nine and older about their evaluation of the program as well as their experiences (the Positive/Negative Experiences Questionnaire and the Rosenberg Self-Esteem Measure). From parents they collect program evaluation ratings as well as information, using the Strengths and Difficulties Questionnaire and the Revised Family Communication Patterns Questionnaire.

- The PATHS program also focuses on children and gathers teacher reports of pre-/post behaviors, peer measures of disruptive versus prosocial behavior in the classroom, and children's reports of their own knowledge and understanding of emotions. The PATHS program has developed a formal evaluation kit that can be used to assess behavior change over time.

- The School Mental Health Team project also focuses on children of soldiers and tracks clinical efforts (case loads, clinical utilization, medication management) and clinical population indicators (e.g., mental health diagnoses, impact of deployment on mental health). They also administer some standard measures (e.g., Strengths and Difficulties Questionnaire) to children and use interactive customer evaluation forms to assess family health and functioning.

- The WRP plans to conduct research on children of deployed and severely injured warriors and will be including in their research studies measures such as the Strengths and Difficulties Questionnaire, Parental Stress Scale, and Survey of Recent Life Experiences, among others.

A number of programs include many different outcomes, consistent with the fact that they are evaluating programs for more than one service and for different populations that they are targeting or because they have more resources to evaluate their programs.

- Battlemind includes satisfaction and attitudinal ratings as well as measures of PTSD, depression, aggressive behaviors/anger, stigma, sleep problems, alcohol problems, work-related attitudes (e.g., Lynch et al., 1999).

- ACEP gathers information on patient satisfaction and knowledge learned during training as well as information on performance-related outcomes, which vary depending on the target population (e.g., rifle marksmanship, physical fitness scores, agility, target specification for marksmanship qualification standards). In addition, ACEP mentioned the use of several published measures (e.g., Kessler's K6 distress measure, CD-RISC, the Sport Anxiety Scale, the State Anxiety Scale, Bartone's Hardiness Measure, the Ottawa assessment tool, Rosenberg's self-esteem scale, the Sport Confidence Inventory, the PTSD Inventory, and the Beck Depression Scale, among others).

- The Marine Resiliency Study (which will be tracking trajectories of adaptation to combat) plans to include an interviewer-administered measure of PTSD, the Peritraumatic Behavior Questionnaire, and the Beck Anxiety and Depression Inventories, as well as a physiologic battery (e.g., startle thresholds, sensory-motor gating, heart rate reactivity) and observer-rated changes in behavior in the aftermath of trauma in their main longitudinal study.
- The PPHDP will assess outcomes of projects at the organizational, individual, and embedded/unit level. They are still developing metrics, but potential outcomes will include psychological health, screening measures, indicators of treatment and counseling patterns, referral and follow-up rates, dropout rates, inpatient hospitalizations, suicide attempts and completions, substance abuse, and workplace, family, and interpersonal violence. Community-based indicators will be incident rates of sexual assault and casualties, as well as family abuse data.

While all programs targeted enhancing some component of resilience (such as hope, well-being, self-esteem, optimism, or personal outlook), relatively few program representatives actually mentioned that they include specific published validated measures of overall "resilience" to monitor program effectiveness.

- In fact, the WRP program representatives mentioned that, in general, resilience measures are limited, especially for children of soldiers.
- ACEP has used the CD-RISC in some studies.
- The new CSF program is using a GAT to monitor soldier performance and resilience in five dimensions: emotional, social, family, spiritual, and physical health.

Because relatively few of the programs have conducted formal evaluations in military populations, there is limited evidence available as to how well the programs are working or would work if they were implemented in the military. We summarize below briefly what each of the programs stated about the impact of their program for military service members and their families.

- ACEP is conducting a number of studies, but results have not yet been published, although the representatives noted that the basic tenets underlying excellence in human performance, which are a feature of their program, should be generalizable to all professions, including the military. In a 2007 assessment of the ACEP program, researchers visited four of nine ACEPs and reviewed their educational protocols. The conclusion was that ACEP fills a gap in the Army's training program and should be institutionalized. ACEP is currently designing studies and mechanisms to provide ongoing assessment and refinement of their curriculum.

- Several studies of the Battlemind program have been published, documenting the extent to which components of their program have been effective. While currently there is no research on the efficacy of in-theater Battlemind psychological debriefing, feedback from military mental health professionals and unit leaders was positive, and the program was rated as helpful by participants and providers (Adler et al., 2009b). Post-deployment Battlemind training has been adapted by the British military and is being evaluated in a group RCT. It is also being integrated into programs in other nations. In a study of Battlemind debriefing and Battlemind training with soldiers returning from Iraq, soldiers with high levels of combat exposure who received Battlemind debriefing reported fewer PTSD and depression symptoms and fewer sleep problems compared with those in a standard stress education program (Adler et al., 2009b). Similarly, soldiers with high levels of combat exposure who received small-group Battlemind training also reported fewer PTSD symptoms and sleep problems compared with stress education participants. Large-group Battlemind training participants with high combat exposure reported fewer PTSD symptoms and lower levels of stigma and—regardless of combat exposure—fewer depression symptoms than did stress education participants. Effect sizes in the high exposure group ranged from 0.20 to 0.30 (in standard deviation units). Basic combat training has been developed by the Walter Reed Army Institute of Research (WRAIR) in conjunction with the Australian Defense Force's BattleSMART program. A pilot study was conducted at Fort Jackson, and a group randomized trial is being conducted as well. Additional studies assessing resilience training that build on the program are being coordinated through WRAIR, while others are being conducted by WRAIR.

- The HeartMath website summarizes a variety of published articles documenting the impact of HeartMath's intervention program. It is only for the past two years that HeartMath has been adapting its program to military populations. Two independent research projects on military populations are in progress. A pilot study of the effect of improving heart rate variability coherence through training in heart rhythm feedback was conducted with five combat veterans who had PTSD. The study found that training resulted in increased total power in heart rate variability, a decrease in false positive responses during a sustained attention task, and improvements in immediate memory. The HeartMath program concluded that it is a promising method for improving deployment-related problems in attention and immediate memory in veterans with PTSD. In addition, HeartMath representatives report that clinicians working with military personnel have stated that the HeartMath system is one of the most effective approaches to helping soldiers improve resiliency and counter the effects of PTSD.

- The developers of the MMFT program conducted a pilot study in 2008 with 35 Marines before deployment to Iraq. Marines completed a battery of behavioral tasks to measure their cognitive capabilities before and after training. Marines who spent more time engaging in MMFT exercises saw an improvement in their cognitive performance. They also maintained their perceived stress level and improved their working memory capacity over their baseline scores. A control group and Marines in the intervention group who practiced fewer mind fitness exercises out of class both saw a decrease in working memory capacity over time. An RCT is now in the planning stages to examine how mind fitness training can build resilience and operational effectiveness among Army soldiers.

- In 2006, the Center for Naval Analyses conducted a pilot of the OSCAR program. The study found that psychologists organic to carrier task forces reduce medical evacuations. One measure of effectiveness is the extent to which the concept of embedding mental health professionals in Marine units has been embraced by Marines. All three Marine expeditionary forces have become enthusiastic about OSCAR, and Marine air wings and logistics groups have requested their own OSCAR teams. The program's success is exemplified by a 97 percent overall return-to-duty rate for all Marines seen in the Marine Expeditionary Force with OSCAR mental health support (Sammons, 2005).

- The Passport Toward Success program collects data from both children and their parents on the day of each event they hold. Overall, they report that ratings of the events are good. Children who reported the most deployment-related stress before the Passport program had the most positive evaluations of the program at the end of the event. Only 10 percent of children said that they had not gotten new ideas for coping with deployment stress during the event. Data collected from parents suggest that the program improves the sense of connection among family members, increases understanding about the benefits of appropriate communication, increases use of coping skills, and increases awareness of emotional needs. Program fidelity data gathered by research observers are also used to evaluate impact. To date, they report 71 percent fidelity across 115 sessions.

- Evidence on the impact of the SMHT is provided by satisfaction ratings and tracking of clinical effort (e.g., symptom presence and severity information is gathered at the initial visits and at the end of three months of treatment or termination). Their resilience programs have shown satisfaction ratings of 4.8 out of 5. On average, clients rated the impact of the service on emotional functioning of family members 4.15 and 4.12 (on a 5-point scale) for the impact of the service on adjustment to deployment of the active-duty parent. Monitoring of clinical outcomes suggests reductions in problem behaviors by 20 percent over three months of treatment. Data indicate clinically important improvements in several domains, as measured by the Strengths and Difficulties Questionnaire over three months of therapy. Total difficulties declined to a more typical range. Satisfaction surveys found that approximately 99 percent were satisfied with the group they attended, and a similar high percentage found the group and material helpful.

- For SLWES, satisfaction surveys were administered by core staff. Participants reported interest in the seminars and looked forward to the topics. As seminars continued, participants became more open and able to discuss their own challenges.

- The SELF program was designed as a clinical screening method to identify and subsequently intervene with soldiers, not as a research project. The impact of the program is evidenced by the fact that the goal of SELF (to guarantee access to behavioral health care) has been met: 100 percent of soldiers who participated in the program have at least one behavioral health follow-up visit. The program identifies new problems and increases the propensity to seek behavioral help. As reported in a 2009 Northwest Guardian report, 41,000 service members at Fort Lewis had completed post-deployment assessments, and 16,000 referrals had been made. The SELF survey provides commanders with information relevant to their unit and allows them to compare their unit with the entire group of soldiers who have been through the program.

- SWTP had several phases in which data were collected primarily by the chaplain who designed and conducted the program. At-risk service members were identified through questionnaires. Those at high risk were given one-on-one confidential attention. During the last weeks of training, information was gathered about the morale of the unit, how soldiers were getting along, and the impact of the unit ministry team on each service member's training. Reports were given to commanders about training, cohesion, and morale of their units.

- WRT was an optional class for soldiers rather than an intervention or a formal Army program. Personal qualitative exit interviews and command letters of support suggested the course's popularity. As of September 2008, over 160 WRT classes with approximately 4,500 participants had been conducted in OIF. Data from an anonymous five-question feedback form suggest positive trends toward WRT acceptance as a class. Written feedback comments suggest that WRT is a beneficial combat stress–control class. WRT was selected as a Suicide Reduction Resiliency initiative used to train 325 WRT instructor trainers in the OIF theater based on consistently positive feedback.

Other programs we reviewed have some evidence of impact but primarily on nonmilitary populations.

- The PRP program has demonstrated its impact in increasing optimism and reducing conduct problems, hopelessness, depression, and anxiety symptoms in children and adolescents. The program, while being modified and tailored for use in a soldier population as part of CSF, does not yet have evidence available for impact in that population.

- Gallup has conducted numerous analyses on its programs with different organizations. They reported that they could develop programs and interventions based on their published tools and robust research findings that could be used in the military to lead to higher levels of engagement at work and in life. They currently have many benchmarks for military clients that could be used as a best-practice database, which would allow Gallup researchers to provide analyses and recommendations.

The evidence above is sparse in terms of showing strong effects of these programs on military resilience. In part, this is due to the fact that such studies require rigorous controlled trials, which have been rare. However, some evidence is being accumulated to support program effectiveness, and several major controlled trials are in the planning or early funding stages. Many of the programs we reviewed stated that they would like to conduct formal evaluations of their programs in the military to support their own assessment of the positive impact of their program.

Future Steps the Programs Would Like to Undertake, Given More Resources

We ended our interviews by asking each program representative what he or she would do differently or additionally related to assessing program effectiveness if more resources were available. Here we summarize some of the relevant themes.

- More robust evaluation:
  - Battlemind is currently submitting proposals to obtain funding to evaluate the program in-theater and in the community, as well as to evaluate their training for leaders and their training for at-risk units post-deployment. They would like to complete validation studies before widespread implementation.
  - The Marine Resiliency Study is in progress. They are looking for additional funding to expand the genetics component of their study and would like to have a longer follow-up period (presently they are conducting assessments one week, three months, and six months post-deployment).
  - With greater resources, the COSC program representatives reported that they would include self-report outcome measures to determine if the program improves readiness, preservation, and health and to address cost-benefit issues. In addition, the program representatives would get feedback from leaders on the benefits of the program and their impressions of the readiness of their force.
  - The OSISS program representatives would develop a performance measure to help them determine an appropriate caseload for peer support coordinators. In addition, program staff are currently working on developing a better screening tool.

- – The Passport Toward Success program representatives would conduct a large-scale RCT to evaluate their program. They are currently identifying strategies for collecting data from locations to do more treatment-as-usual projects. In addition, the program representatives would construct and study a continual process that builds skills, strengthens skills, and continues with post-deployment programming components. They would plan to track children as they get older and follow families over time.
- – The PATHS program is being tailored to the military context. The representatives would like to be able to include long-term follow-up to their programs and would look at outcomes of children during the high school years.
- – The School Mental Health Team noted the need for a validated measure of soldier readiness.
- – With additional resources, the SELF program representatives would add additional population-normed instruments to the Post-Deployment Health Reassessment Program (PDHRA) to screen for additional areas of concern. In addition, while initially conceptualized as a clinical event to help soldiers, research is needed to determine the advantages of SWAP/SELF relative to the standard PDHRA process to facilitate a cost-benefit analysis. For example, the developers of this program would plan to conduct a random-assignment controlled trail of SELF compared with treatment as usual or a pre-SELF/post-SELF study looking at utilization of behavioral health care, stigma, and satisfaction.
- – The WRP representatives would like to see more emphasis on development and validations of resilience measures for children. WRT representatives would also have their program formally evaluated. Given additional resources, the WRT program representatives would compare their program with units exposed to other psychological education programs.
- Dissemination of resilience training programs to other types of settings and organizations:
  - – Trials are needed with Guard or Reserve members (e.g., the Employee Engagement Program, which would like to better prove the case for taking their program into intact organizations).
  - – The HeartMath group has been adapting its program for military populations over the past two years. They would plan to take training to military families at the community level. They feel that community-level resilience is the missing component from the military perspective. HeartMath would like to shift the focus from bases or units to communities.
  - – The JSB would put additional focus on mental illness prevention efforts by teaching skills to foster resilience early on and developing the curriculum to be delivered at recruitment through the end of the deployment spectrum. They would also like to get family and the community more involved in the program.
- Hiring and training more staff:

- The Employee Engagement Program representatives would train trainers for all their major hubs and satellite locations worldwide.
- JSB representatives would increase the involvement of credible people who would be leveraged within the program.
- Landing Gear representatives expressed a desire for additional personnel and time for training.
- The MMFT program representatives would continue collecting longitudinal data, since it is difficult to assess resilience over short time periods with the kinds of psychological injuries that soldiers are experiencing.
- The SWTP representative would develop training for other chaplains and focus on training in the area of resiliency. Additional resources would also be used to find more personnel to help manage the spiritual needs of soldiers; develop a more formal program with administrative staff, workbooks, trainers, and students; move the program into U.S. Army Forces Command units; and develop an enhanced leadership skills development program.
- WRT representatives would also take more time to train and would like to be given the opportunity to present more information about WRT so that it might be adopted as a formal Army program.

- More follow-up activities after initial training:
  - With more resources, the Energy Project would ask every organization to conduct an organizational energy audit. They would design follow-on activities that would allow clients to reengage with the program material. Ideally, they would like to be able to spend time with a team in order to witness interactions and help individuals apply program principles in real time.
  - Gallup would provide additional interventions to increase engagement and improve unit performance. These could include additional education, training, and impact planning on the Q-12 and Hope instruments. The result would be improved performance outcomes, including increased control, stability, and peer support, which will lead to improved resilience capacity. Gallup would also conduct additional consulting, training, and coaching for leaders, commanders, and supervisors. Additional performance-impact analyses could include linking engagement to the familial setting and the community at large.
  - MMFT representatives would develop a maintenance training course that goes beyond the unit training.

- Further program curriculum development:
  - Landing Gear is currently being revised to make it more performance-based (e.g., performance enhancement, reassurance, and encouragement). In addition, representatives said they would further develop their Wingman online material and encourage more people to use it. They are in the process of planning a more targeted system in which those airmen who are symptomatic are provided extra information and services in a more proactive manner.

- The National Guard Resiliency Program is developing a family course curriculum with service members and their wives or husbands and children. Additional resources would allow them to coordinate the many different resiliency programs that are being conducted in many states. They would then identify successful programs rather than build new programs from scratch. Presently, the National Guard Resiliency Program trains 39 days a year in the National Guard. They would like to include aspects of the CSF program in their training. They would also use further funding to support continued training programs, with the goal of moving from the state to the national level.

Overall, the program staff we interviewed wanted opportunities to improve on their programs and establish their effectiveness in order to become more widespread in the military context.

CHAPTER FOUR

Conclusions and Recommendations

This monograph sought to identify the factors that promote resilience by reviewing evidence available in the literature. Although the factors were not empirically derived, they were gathered using a rigorous qualitative approach. They were then used to examine a subset of programs designed to promote resilience in military populations, in order to better understand which evidence-informed factors are utilized by those programs. This chapter summarizes the study's main findings and reviews recommended actions that can be taken by those currently implementing resilience programs, those planning to develop new programs, and policymakers seeking to improve services and maintain readiness by enhancing well-being among military members and their families.

Conclusions

Our review of the resilience literature and review of selected programs designed to promote resilience led to several conclusions. We organize these conclusions in four parts:

1. factors that promote resilience
2. assessments of program effectiveness
3. barriers to program implementation
4. implications for further work on resilience.

Factors That Promote Resilience

The literature review identified a set of factors that are supported by evidence in the literature and by a group of academic experts in the resilience field (some of whom have military experience). The factors are presented based on the level at which they operate: individual, family, unit, or community (see p. xiv for detailed descriptions of factors).

- Individual-level factors
  - Positive coping
  - Positive affect
  - Positive thinking

- – Realism
- – Behavioral control
- Family-level factors
  - – Emotional ties
  - – Communication
  - – Support
  - – Closeness
  - – Nurturing
  - – Adaptability
- Unit-level factors
  - – Positive command climate
  - – Teamwork
  - – Cohesion
- Community-level factors
  - – Belongingness
  - – Cohesion
  - – Connectedness
  - – Collective efficacy

Based on findings from the literature review, there was stronger scientific evidence for individual- and unit-level factors, though generally very little rigorous research is available across factors—only 11 of the 270 documents that we reviewed employed a randomized control design. The individual resilience factors that had moderate evidence (based on cross-sectional correlational or observational design) or strong evidence (based on an RCT or longitudinal design) were positive thinking, positive affect, positive coping, realism, and behavioral control. Family social support had the most evidence among the family-level factors. For unit-level factors, positive command climate had the most evidence, and at the community level, belongingness had the most evidence. The stronger the scientific evidence, the more important the factor in promoting resilience.

The 23 programs that we reviewed were purposefully selected to illustrate a variety of resilience content, target audiences, and applications to the military. Most of the programs addressed psychological content (as opposed to physical, social, or spiritual) and were targeted to either military members or families of military members. The programs addressed all phases of the deployment cycle. Most programs primarily offered workshops or classes, though other forms of service delivery were also provided.

A number of important themes emerged regarding the role of these resilience factors in programs and the barriers experienced in delivering the programs. Individual- and unit-level factors were the most commonly incorporated resilience factors across programs. Consistent with the literature review, we found that most program materials employ some form of positive thinking, positive coping, behavioral control, positive affect, and realism training at the individual level. A majority of programs also incorporate positive command climate (which had a good deal of evidence) and teamwork (with less evidence) at the unit level. Among the family-level factors, enhancing communication and support were also relatively widely employed approaches to promoting resilience. Increasing belongingness had the most evidence from the literature review and was also the most common factor among programs promoting community resilience.

Since strength is already an inherent value within the military culture, promoting psychological resilience as a form of strength is a natural fit. Therefore, additional resilience training programs that are incorporated into existing strength training structures are likely to be promising.

Assessing Program Effectiveness at Promoting Resilience

Consistent with the many different resilience programs, there was great variability in the measures they used to gauge their effectiveness. At the individual level, measures commonly used to evaluate program effectiveness were mental health–related, implying that resilience is defined in terms of absence of mental health symptoms or conditions such as PTSD, depression, anxiety, and anger. However, others included measures of well-being, positive affect, self-regulation, and mindfulness, reflecting a strengths-based focus. Others focused on performance and functioning, either in general (e.g., using the GAT) or for targeted populations (e.g., increased productivity for workers, return to duty or reduced training failures for soldiers). At the family, unit, and community levels, a variety of other measures were used to assess effectiveness of the programs that targeted those populations, including family satisfaction, family communication patterns, unit engagement, and perceived organizational support. No standard measures of resilience or outcomes are used across resilience programs.

Barriers to Program Implementation

There were five types of barriers to implementation and program operation commonly identified by the representatives of resilience programs we reviewed. The most prevalent barrier to program success was lack of support from military leadership. Other barriers included logistical challenges associated with coordinating training efforts and program events in the context of a dynamic and demanding military environment. Limited funding was also mentioned as a barrier to sustainment and expansion of many resilience programs, particularly with regard to bridging mental health and military training paradigms—neither of which are fully aligned with resilience paradigms. Several programs also mentioned the challenges of tailoring program content to the military audience and the stigma of mental health. Despite these barriers, many programs were able to overcome them. Some of the primary lessons were to involve senior leadership early in the program development process, adopt a flexible curriculum, and reorient the content to emphasize strength building and similarity to physical fitness.

Few of the programs we reviewed have conducted and published RCTs or other rigorously designed studies to establish program effectiveness in military populations. However, those that have include Battlemind, ACEP, HeartMath, and PRP. Additionally, several programs are in the planning stages of evaluation (Marine Resiliency Study, MMFT, OSCAR, and PPHDP). Most programs have been implemented before evidence of their effectiveness has been established. Programs often are modified for each client or context, making it difficult to design studies that will provide evidence of effectiveness for all military populations and situations. New scientific studies have recently been funded and are in the planning or initial data collection stages, but, as with most quasi-experimental or controlled studies, it will be a number of years before evidence of their effectiveness is fully established. As these studies with evaluative data progress, they should be encouraged to publish their results.

Implications for Further Work on Resilience

Ideally, to select the most promising resilience programs, it would be helpful to develop standardized resilience measures that could be applied to a variety of populations in different contexts and allow for comparison among programs. Such measures would incorporate some of the factors, such as positive affect, positive coping, realism, behavioral control, family social support, and positive command climate (at the individual, family, unity and community level), that we identified during our literature review. While our review did not include an evaluation of resilience measures themselves there are a number of published resilience scales (e.g., the CD-RISC Scale, Brief Resilient Coping Scale, and Resilience Scale for Adults [Connor and Davidson, 2003; Friborg et al., 2003; and Sinclair and Wallston, 2004]), general measures of psychological well-being (e.g., Ryff and Keyes, 1995, documents a measure of psychological well-being that encompasses six dimensions of wellness: autonomy, environmental realism, personal growth, positive relations with others, purpose in life, and self-acceptance), and factor-specific scales (e.g., Rosenberg self-esteem scale [Rosenberg, 1965]). Adult measures of factor- or content-specific scales (such as positive coping styles, optimism, hope, sense of control, self-esteem, autonomy, and spirituality) are summarized in Snyder and Lopez's 2006 book on positive psychological assessment.

Given the lack of consensus on what factors promote resilience, the fact that there is no single agreed-on measure to assess resilience, and the fact that existing measures were developed and validated primarily with nonmilitary populations, further methodological development of resilience scales for the military is warranted. A detailed review of resilience measures and the extent to which they are valid for military members and their families would be valuable. However, given the potentially large number of published instruments from which to choose and the potential respondent burden associated with measuring so many resilience factors, it may be worth developing a new resilience measure, based on the overall conceptual structure and list of factors, that is reliable and valid for military populations and their families. For example, as part of the Army's CSF program, a GAT that provides information on four dimensions of strength (emotional, social, spiritual, and family) is being developed (CSF-GAT). The extent to which it covers all important resilience factors will be important to determine, along with its generalizability to the other services. Similar measures for families of service members should also be developed for those programs that focus on families and children.

Study Strengths and Limitations

This study fills some gaps in knowledge about which factors promote resilience, with particular attention to how to do so in military populations, but still has some limitations. With regard to the literature review, we did not look at all of the available articles and other written documents. This literature is extremely far-ranging, and to do a completely comprehensive survey of all resilience literature would have been beyond the scope of this study. Instead, we targeted and bounded the search to capture the bolus of the literature published from 2000 to the present. Most of our search covered the period until spring 2009, but we did add materials that were provided by the programs we reviewed in the six-month period following the database search. Rather than summarizing all the documents using a traditional literature review format, we targeted the reviews so that for each document we honed in on factors that promote resilience, using a standardized abstraction form to maximize the consistency across reviewers. While we did not formally assess inter-rater reliability, we did use a pile-sort approach to code the resilience factors and group discussion to resolve inconsistencies, which strengthened our consistency across the team. In addition, our review focused on psychological resilience and, therefore, did not include other important factors (e.g., nutrition and other health behaviors, such as getting adequate sleep and moderating alcohol use) that may influence "total fitness," a concept that the Department of Defense is emphasizing for the military population. These factors are important aspects of resilience, but it was beyond the scope of the study for such a broad literature review.

Another limitation of the literature review is that evidence ratings, by nature, are subjective. We tried to minimize any subjectivity by having the three evidence raters discuss how they interpreted the criteria for determining the scores (none, weak, moderate, or strong). A series of four one-hour meetings to discuss the ratings were conducted. Where there were inconsistencies, the team agreed on resolutions and incorporated those decisions into subsequent factor ratings.

There are four limitations related to our program review. First, we could not review the entire sample of programs that attempt to promote resilience and, thus, purposefully selected a subset particularly applicable to the military. Without a random selection of programs, we may have missed the opportunity to learn about other types of programming to promote resilience that are not reflected in our review.

Another limitation of our program review is the possibility of socially desirable responses from program representatives, especially with regard to their reports about specific resilience factors associated with their respective programs. The information on resilience factors featured in the reviewed programs is based on a combination of information gleaned from program documents and interviews. In some cases, program representatives indicated that a factor is part of the program, but we did not obtain concrete documentation of how the factor is part of training or education. In other cases, the factor was identified as promoting resilience by the program as a secondary element of the program rather than as a driving force. Thus, interviewees may have had a tendency to give the answers they believed the interviewer wanted to hear.

In addition, semi-structured interviews are by nature biased because it is often unclear how to interpret missing information. For example, just because a topic is not mentioned by the interviewee, it is not necessarily the case that it was not addressed by the program.

Finally, some individuals have different styles of conversing so that some are able to cover more information than others within the allotted time for the interview.

Policy Recommendations

Based on our analyses, we offer a series of recommendations for those responsible for developing or implementing resilience programs within the military. These are outlined below:

Define Resilience

As our study shows, there are a variety of definitions of resilience in the literature, making a summary of the field difficult. We chose a definition that encapsulates both the concept of capacity and the concept of a process involving adaptation and experiencing stressful situations. Our definition also conceptualizes outcomes in a positive orientation (psychological health and strength) rather than a negative one (mental illness and weakness), which is more amenable to the military context. Senior commanders and policymakers should carefully formulate a definition of resilience that reflects both the literature and the military culture as a necessary first step in building any existing programs. A clear definition will not only clarify program stakeholders' understanding of their mission but will also provide clear guidance for those developing program outcome measures.

Integrate Resilience into Policy and Doctrine

To implement resilience programs effectively, the DoD should consider clear policy to define resilience, to assign roles and responsibilities across the services, and to provide guidance on program implementation. Since building resilience is largely a function of focused training, such policy could identify the Under Secretary of Defense (USD) for Personnel and Readiness as the prime oversight organization for training, implementation, and monitoring. The USD for Personnel and Readiness is the most logical oversight organization because most resilience researchers are behavioral scientists, whose work would normally inform the military health system; placing responsibility for resilience programs in Health Affairs, however, could possibly hamper implementation of resilience initiatives by operational commanders. Good policy would clearly identify the main factors in building resilience, would properly align oversight with personnel programs, and would allow for flexible implementation that reflects the unique culture of each of the services.

Strengthen Existing Resilience Programs

While several of the programs we reviewed have proven effective in promoting resilience in military groups, others have not had the resources or opportunity to evaluate program success, and, therefore, their value is uncertain. Military commanders will only endorse programs that add value to already-busy training schedules. Without data to demonstrate their value, further investments in programming will be hard to sell. More formal evaluations will help to identify strengths and weaknesses of existing programs, possibly aligning the resilience factors identified here. In addition, pilot studies using RCTs to compare programs with the strongest available evidence (e.g., the CSF program's effort to develop robust comparisons) are recommended. However, we do acknowledge the difficulties in designing RCTs for military populations, given the need to address resilience concerns for all members, not only for random samples. Thus, comparative effectiveness studies, randomized studies with wait list controls, and other creative designs may be necessary to consider.

The DCoE is ideally positioned to serve as a clearinghouse for researching and marketing resilience programs, and the military services are encouraged to use their staff as a central resource. Not only do they have a variety of outreach tools and services, they also have a fully staffed Resilience Directorate. Although individual service requirements may vary, making resilience programs slightly different among the services, the DCoE is resourced and staffed to coordinate research efforts, to disseminate best practices, and to consult as needed to program implementation offices. In addition, they can readily identify those programs with the most promise for using evidence-based approaches to building resilience.

Standardize Resilience Measures to Enable Program Comparisons

As noted above, developing standardized measures for use with the military would be an important contribution to understanding the success of resilience-building programs. Such measures would incorporate evidence-based factors from the study framework and could build on or adapt existing resilience measures and related measures of the resilience factors. Such an effort would move the field toward consensus about what factors comprise resilience, which measure is most valid and reliable for assessing resilience, and their relevance for military populations. This would entail a detailed review of resilience measures and the development of a new resilience measure based on the overall conceptual structure and list of factors that are reliable and valid for military populations and their families. The GAT being developed for the Army is a step in this direction. Similar measures for families and children are needed. Another approach to consider is to develop a comprehensive item bank for measuring resilience, using the principles of item response theory (IRT) to support the development of short-form measures and computer adaptive testing to address issues of respondent burden and comparability across populations.

Provide Military Members and Their Families Guidance About the Different Resilience Programs Available

With the rapid increase in the number of resilience programs available, it may be difficult for individuals to decipher the advantages of various programs. A resource guide for resilience programs that compares and contrasts the different types of services offered by different programs would serve to increase awareness about different options. Such a guide should also include any evidence on the programs' effects. Again, this would be an excellent project for the DCoE to undertake on behalf of the Services.

Incorporate Evidence-Based Resilience Factors

New programs designed to promote resilience should incorporate factors with the most evidence. Thus, the military community will benefit most from programs that teach individuals (military members, family members of military, and leaders) techniques that enhance positive affect, positive thinking, coping, realism, and behavioral control. At the family level, programs that bolster support, communication, and nurturing are likely to be the most beneficial. Group-level factors that have the most benefit are positive command climate and belongingness. Thus, programs that train military leaders to build realism and confidence among their troops are recommended, and efforts to engage all members of the military community by providing opportunities to participate in integrated activities will likely promote resilience.

Adopt a Flexible Curriculum

Resilience programs must be designed to dovetail with existing training and community-based programs. At the individual and unit levels, regularly scheduled training should include materials that capture the factors described in this monograph. While subject matter experts might be used to develop the training materials, actual training should be delivered alongside existing operational training. An excellent example of this is the Marine OSCAR program, which delivers resilience concepts in a format already familiar to Marines. Similarly, programs designed to promote family and community resilience should use existing structures and programs already in place in the community. Chapel and family programs already offer ideal structures, venues, and staff to deliver resilience training—and, in fact, many of the programs reviewed are currently being offered through military family and community programs and staff.

Engage Senior Military Leaders

As discussed in Chapter Three, a major challenge to building a resilience program within the military culture is getting support from senior operational leadership. Not only should oversight of resilience programs be placed in personnel training programs, but operational commanders must also fully understand their role in building a resilient force. It is especially important to design programs with the involvement of senior military leaders in order to motivate service members' interest by promoting values that are important to the service cultures. It is vital that operational commanders be involved in promoting resilience programs and in creating conditions that ensure participation in programs. Without strong leadership, military resilience programs cannot be successful. As an example, the Real Warriors Campaign to combat stigma features prominent military leaders who actively participate in and promote the program. Service career schools for training leaders, such as the Marine Corps University and the Army's Command and Staff College, are a means for promoting resilience among service members.

Conduct More Rigorous Program Evaluation

Although there are many programs available to the military and civilian communities, there is very little empirical evidence that these programs effectively build resilience. Similarly, there are a number of factors related to resilience, but there is almost no evidence that resilience can be taught or produced. Results from both the literature review and the program review echo the need for more program evaluation, as identified as one of the missions of the DCoE. As noted, only 11 documents in the literature review are based on RCT evaluation design, and only five of the programs reviewed have formally evaluated program success, yet programs are often rolled out before evidence of their effectiveness has been established and are modified for each client or context, making it difficult to provide evidence for effectiveness across populations and situations. In general, studies of resilience in the military should enhance scientific rigor by conducting more RCTs and longitudinal studies that span the phases of deployment. This is particularly true for military families, since little research has been published in this area (MacDermid et al., 2008). In addition, studies with existing evaluative data need to be encouraged to publish their results.

Conclusion

Promoting resilience in the military is an increasingly important objective of DoD. Effective programs that improve service members and their families' resilience directly assist the military in keeping its personnel better prepared for combat. Our study reached the following conclusions:

- There is evidence in the literature supporting many factors that can help to promote resilience at the individual, family, unit, and community levels.
  - Scientific evidence is especially strong for positive thinking, positive affect, positive coping, realism, and behavioral control, as well as for positive command climate and belongingness.
- Many of the programs that were reviewed as part of this study incorporate these evidence-based factors into their core missions.
- However, interviews with program representatives identified five types of challenges to program implementation, which suggest opportunities to improve program capabilities:
  - lack of leadership support by the military
  - problems with logistics
  - limited funding to sustain programs
  - poor fit within the military culture
  - mental health stigma.

Building resilience in the military can be strengthened in several ways. Clear policy to define roles, responsibilities, and broad guidance for implementation would be extremely helpful. Using evidence-based resilience factors in a flexible, culturally sensitive context is also important. Resilience policies should also direct more rigorous program evaluation, using standardized measures and comparing across different programs. Such evaluations could help guide military members and their families to make informed decisions about program selection. Ultimately, strong command leadership will enable the success of resilience programming and will enhance the overall strength and resilience of service members and their families.

Summary of Definitions

Table A.1
General Resilience Definitions

Definition	Source	Basic/ Adaptation/ Growth
"A complex repertoire of behavioral tendencies"	Agaibi and Wilson (2005)	Basic
"A style of behavior with identifiable patterns of thinking, perceiving, and decisionmaking across different types of situations"	Agaibi and Wilson (2005)	Basic
"The ability to maintain a state of normal equilibrium in the face of extremely unfavorable circumstances"	Ahmed (2007)	Adaptation
"The dynamic process of transactions within and among multiple levels of children's environment over time that influences their capacity to successfully adapt and function despite experiencing chronic stress and adversity"	Aisenberg and Herrenkohl (2008)	Adaptation
"The capacity to develop a high degree of competence in spite of stressful environments and experiences"	Allison et al. (2003)	Adaptation
"The ability to recover from or adjust easily to misfortune or sustained life stress"	Allison et al. (2003)	Adaptation
"Positive outcomes in the face of adversity"	Alriksson-Schmidt (2007)	Adaptation
"Successful adaptation despite risk and adversity. Resilience requires exposure to significant risks, overcoming risks or adversity, and success that is beyond predicted expectations."	Barton (2003)	Growth
"The hardy-resilient style is a generalized mode of functioning that incorporates a strong sense of commitment and meaning in life, an expectation that one can control or influence outcomes, and an adventurous, exploring approach to living."	Bartone et al. (2009)	Basic
"Emergence over time of unexpected strengths and competencies in those at risk"	Beardslee (2002)	Growth

Table A.1—Continued

Definition	Source	Basic/ Adaptation/ Growth
". . . (a) having curiosity and intellectual mastery; (b) having compassion—with detachment; (c) having the ability to conceptualize; (d) obtaining the conviction of one's right to survive; (e) possessing the ability to remember and invoke images of good and sustaining figures; (f) having the ability to be in touch with affects, not denying or suppressing major affects as they arise; (g) having a goal to live for; (h) having the ability to attract and use support; (i) possessing a vision of the possibility and desirability of restoration civilized moral order; (j) having the need and ability to help others; (k) having an affective repertory; (l) being resourceful; (m) being altruistic toward others; and (o) having the capacity to turn traumatic helplessness into learned helpfulness"	Bell (2001)	Basic
"Characteristics, dimensions, and properties of families which help families to be resistant to disruption in the face of change, and adaptive in the face of crisis situations"	Black and Lobo (2008) and Patterson (2002)	Adaptation
"The ability of adults in otherwise normal circumstances who are exposed to an isolated/and potentially highly disruptive event . . . to maintain relatively stable, healthy levels of psychological functioning."	Bonanno et al. (2007)	Adaptation
"Resilient individuals . . . generally exhibit a stable trajectory of healthy functioning across time, as well as the capacity for generative experiences and positive emotions."	Bonanno (2004)	Adaptation
"The ability to maintain a stable equilibrium"	Bonanno (2004)	Basic
"Not only the ability to rapidly 'bounce back' in the aftermath of inescapable extreme adversities, such as large-scale natural disasters, terrorist attacks, or warzone exposure, but also the quality of being 'unflappable' during the event or even to feel strengthened by it."	Bracha and Bienvenu (2005)	Growth
"The processes underlying successful adaptation under adverse conditions"	Butler et al. (2007)	Adaptation
"The capacity to cope with or adapt to significant risk and adversity and to recover quickly from stressful change or misfortune"	Campbell et al. (2008)	Adaptation
"The homeostatic return to a prior condition"	Carver (1998)	Basic
"An enduring characteristic of the person, a situational or temporal interaction between the person and the context, or a unitary or multifaceted construct, and it can be applied to social, academic, or other settings."	Condly (2006)	Basic
"Success in meeting tasks and expectations"	Condly (2006)	Basic
"The maintenance and orientation of homeostasis and functionally optimal adaptation"	Condly (2006)	Adaptation
"The ability to thrive in the face of obstacles or adverse circumstances"	Condly (2006)	Growth

Table A.1—Continued

Definition	Source	Basic/ Adaptation/ Growth
"The intersection of a child w/ trauma or a toxic environment in which success is achieved by virtue of the child's abilities, motivations, and support systems"	Condly (2006)	Adaptation
"A dynamic process encompassing positive adaptation within the context of significant adversity"	Conger and Conger (2002); Coleman and Ganong (2002); and Luthar, Cicchetti, and Becker (2000)	Adaptation
"The personal qualities that enable one to thrive in the face of adversity"	Connor and Davidson (2003)	Growth
"A multidimensional characteristic that varies with context, time, age, gender, and cultural origin, as well as within an individual subjected to different life circumstances"	Connor and Davidson (2003)	Basic
"A measure of stress-coping ability . . . it describes personal qualities that allow individuals and communities to grow and even thrive in the face of adversity."	Connor (2006)	Growth
"An improved or enhanced adaptive outcome"	Earvolino-Ramirez (2007)	Growth
"The ability to bounce back or cope successfully despite substantial adversity"	Earvolino-Ramirez (2007)	Adaptation
"The process of overcoming the negative effects of risk exposure, coping successfully with traumatic experiences, and avoiding the negative trajectories associated with risks"	Fergus and Zimmerman (2005, p. 399)	Adaptation
"Resilient individuals are said to bounce back from stressful experiences quickly and efficiently, just as resilient metals bend but do not break. Relative to their less resilient peers, resilient individuals exhibit faster cardiovascular recovery following a high-activation negative emotion."	Fredrickson (2001)	Adaptation
"A relatively stable personality trait characterized by the ability to bounce back from negative experience and by flexible adaptation to the ever-changing demands of life"	Fredrickson et al. (2003)	Adaptation
"[Resilient individuals] sustain normal development despite long-term stress, adversity, or maltreatment."	Friborg et al. (2006)	Adaptation
"A universal capacity which allows a person, group, or community to prevent, minimize, or overcome the damaging effects of adversity"	Ghazinour (2003)	Adaptation
"The ability to successfully adapt to stressors, maintaining psychological well-being in the face of adversity"	Haglund et al. (2007)	Adaptation
"A class of phenomena characterized by patterns of positive adaptation in the context of significant adversity or loss"	Hart (2006)	Adaptation

Table A.1—Continued

Definition	Source	Basic/ Adaptation/ Growth
"A dynamic process influenced by protective factors, conceptualized as the specific skills and abilities necessary for the process of resilience to occur"	Hart (2006)	Basic
"The presence of protective factors that buffer effects of adversity"	Hjemdal et al. (2006)	Adaptation
"A good outcome despite experiencing situations that carry a sufficient risk for developing psychopathology"	Hjemdal et al. (2006)	Adaptation
"[Resilience] encompasses psychological and biological characteristics, intrinsic to an individual, that might be modifiable and that confer protection against the development of psychopathology in the face of stress."	Hoge et al. (2007)	Adaptation
"Resilient individuals are those who experience a trauma but do not develop PTSD."	Hoge et al. (2007)	Adaptation
"Resilient families are able to adapt and continue to function well during mobilization and deployments and they are able to meet other challenges of military duty and family life."	Huebner and Mancini (2005)	Adaptation
"One's capacity to adapt successfully in the presence of risk and adversity"	Jensen and Fraser (2005)	Adaptation
"An ability to recover from or adjust easily to misfortune or change"	Laraway (2007)	Adaptation
"The product of dynamic interactions between a range of risk and protective factors internal and external to a person at various stages of a person's life"	Lepore and Revenson (2006)	Basic
"A multidimensional construct that encompasses a variety of adaptive processes and outcomes. Resilience is evident when individuals are able to resist and recover from stressful situations, or reconfigure their thoughts, beliefs, and behaviors to adjust to ongoing and changing demands."	Lepore and Revenson (2006)	Adaptation
"Dynamic processes that lead to adaptive outcomes in the face of adversity"	Lepore and Revenson (2006)	Adaptation
"[Resilience] is more than just a personality trait; it is the product of the person, his or her past experiences, and current life context."	Lepore and Revenson (2006)	Basic
"A process or capacity that develops over time in the context of person-environmental interactions"	Letourneau et al. (2001)	Basic
"The ability to bounce back from negative emotional experiences and by flexible adaptation to the changing demands of stressful experiences"	Litz (2007) and Tugade and Fredrickson (2004)	Adaptation
"The positive end of the distribution of developmental outcomes among individuals at high risk"	Luthar and Cicchetti (2000)	Growth

Table A.1—Continued

Definition	Source	Basic/ Adaptation/ Growth
"At-risk individuals show better-than-expected outcomes."	Luthar and Cicchetti (2000)	Adaptation
"Positive adaptation is maintained despite the occurrence of stressful experiences."	Luthar and Cicchetti (2000)	Adaptation
"There is a good recovery from trauma."	Luthar and Cicchetti (2000)	Adaptation
"A dynamic process wherein individuals display positive adaptation despite experiences of significant adversity or trauma"	Luthar and Cicchetti (2000)	Adaptation
"[Resilience involves] a developmental progression such that new vulnerabilities and/or strengths often emerge with changing life circumstances."	Luthar et al. (2000)	Growth
"Exposure to adverse or traumatic circumstances [and] successful adaptation following exposure"	MacDermid et al. (2008)	Adaptation
"A dynamic developmental process driven by the interactions among risk and protective factors at an interpersonal and environmental level"	Maeseele et al. (2008)	Basic
"Growth and positive life changes that may result from exposure to traumatic incidents"	Maguen et al. (2006)	Growth
"Flexibility in the face of ever-changing situational demands, including the ability to recover from negative and stressful experiences and find positive meaning in seemingly adverse situations"	Maguen et al. (2008)	Adaptation
"The capacity for generative experiences and positive emotions"	Mancini and Bonanno (2006)	Basic
"The capacity to maintain healthy, symptom-free functioning following a potentially traumatic event"	Mancini and Bonanno (2006)	Adaptation
"The ability of adults in otherwise normal circumstances who are exposed to an isolated and potentially highly disruptive event such as the death of a close relation or violent or life-threatening situation to maintain relatively stable, healthy levels of psychological and physical functioning"	Mancini and Bonanno (2006) and Bonanno (2004)	Adaptation
"A common phenomenon arising from ordinary human adaptive processes"	Masten (2001)	Basic
"A class of phenomena characterized by good outcomes in spite of serious threats to adaptation or development"	Masten (2001)	Adaptation
"Adapting well in the face of adversity"	Meichenbaum (2006)	Adaptation
"Resistance to and rapid recovery from psychiatric illness"	Nemeroff et al. (2006)	Adaptation

Table A.1—Continued

Definition	Source	Basic/ Adaptation/ Growth
"The ability of an individual, a group, an organization, or even an entire population to rapidly and effectively rebound from psychological perturbations associated with critical incidents, terrorism, and even mass disasters"	Nucifora et al. (2007)	Adaptation
"Bouncing back from traumatic experiences"	Nucifora et al. (2007)	Adaptation
"Bounding back through adversity"	Paton et al. (2003)	Adaptation
"Doing well in the face of adversity"	Patterson (2002)	Adaptation
"The ability to go through difficulties and regain satisfactory quality of life"	Peres et al. (2007)	Adaptation
"The ability to adjust to stress and to restore equilibrium when confronted with trauma, tragedy, and threat"	Pfefferbaum et al. (2008)	Adaptation
"A life-sustaining process that must be continued over time and that facilitates growth . . . [and] involves attitudes, behaviors, and skills that can be cultivated, taught, and practiced"	Pfefferbaum et al. (2008)	Basic
"The ability to execute different and effective adjustment processes to alleviate stress and restore equilibrium in the face of trauma, tragedy and threat"	Pfefferbaum et al. (2007)	Adaptation
"An ongoing process involving attitudes, beliefs, and behaviors and even physical functioning that must be sustained over time and support growth"	Pfefferbaum et al. (2007)	Basic
"Individual and family characteristics that explain why somebody not only escapes adversity unscratched, but also blossoms"	Punamaki et al. (2006)	Growth
"The process of adapting well in the face of adversity, trauma, tragedy, threats, or even significant sources of stress"	Ritchie et al. (2006) and Yehuda et al. (2006)	Adaptation
"Post traumatic growth"	Rosner and Powell (2006)	Growth
"Resistance to psychosocial risk experiences"	Rutter (1999)	Adaptation
"The phenomenon of overcoming stress or adversity"	Rutter (1999)	Adaptation
"The capacity to cope with pressure and not break down"	Shalev and Errera (2008)	Adaptation
"The absence of an expected bad outcome, such as general distress, depression, or post-traumatic stress disorder (PTSD)"	Shalev and Errera (2008)	Basic
"An initial loss of functioning and subsequent recovery"	Shalev and Errera (2008)	Basic

Table A.1—Continued

Definition	Source	Basic/ Adaptation/ Growth
"The ability to overcome stress and maintain an effective level of appropriate behavior or performance when confronted by obstacles, setbacks, distractions, hostile conditions, or aversive stimuli"	Staal et al. (2008)	Adaptation
"Being able to learn and adapt"	Stanley (2009)	Basic
"The process of cognitive adaptation to threat . . . restores many people to their prior level of functioning and inspires others to find new meaning in their lives."	Taylor (1983)	Growth
"Bouncing back from life difficulties"	Tedeschi and Calhoun (2003)	Adaptation
"An ability to go on with life after hardship and adversity or to continue living a purposeful life after experiencing hardship and adversity"	Tedeschi and Calhoun (2004)	Adaptation
"Effective coping and adaptation in the face of major life stress"	Tedeschi and Kilmer (2005)	Adaptation
"A combination of abilities and characteristics that interact dynamically to allow an individual to 'bounce back' ('plasticity'), cope successfully, and function above the norm in spite of significant stress or adversity"	Tusaie and Dyer (2004)	Growth
"Both a child's state of well-being and the characteristics and processes by which that well-being is achieved and sustained"	Ungar and Terem (2003)	Basic
"Deployment resilience is the ability to resist the stress of deployment."	Van Breda (2001)	Adaptation
"The strengths that people and systems demonstrate that enable them to rise above or recover from adversity"	Van Breda (2008)	Growth
"Key processes that enable families to cope more effectively and emerge hardier from crises or persistent stresses"	Van Breda (2008)	Growth
"The processes that help adults bounce back from significant negative emotional events"	Van Vliet (2008)	Adaptation
"The achievement of successful adaptation following a period of maladaption or developmental difficulty"	Van Vliet (2008)	Adaptation
"The ability to adapt and successfully cope with adversity, life stressors, and traumatic events"	Wald et al. (2006)	Adaptation
"The human ability to adapt in the face of tragedy, trauma, adversity, hardship, and ongoing significant life stressors"	Wald et al. (2006)	Adaptation
"The capacity to recover or bounce back, as is inherent in its etymological origins, wherein 'resilience' derives from the Latin words salire (to leap or jump), and resilire (to spring back)"	Wald et al. (2006)	Adaptation
"The ability to withstand and rebound from disruptive life challenges"	Walsh (2003)	Adaptation

Table A.1—Continued

Definition	Source	Basic/ Adaptation/ Growth
"The ability to stretch (like elastic) or flex (like a suspension bridge) in response to the pressures and strains of life"	Wiens and Boss (2006)	Adaptation
"The ability to bounce back to a level of functioning equal to or greater than before"	Wiens and Boss (2006)	Growth

Table A.2
Community Resilience Definitions

Definition	Source	Basic/ Adaptation/ Growth
"For a community to be resilient, its members must put into practice early and effective actions so that they can respond to adversity in a healthy manner."	Gurwitch et al. (2007)	Adaptation
"After an event, a [resilient] community may not only be able to cope and recover, but . . . it may also change to reflect different priorities arising from a disaster."	Gurwitch et al. (2007)	Growth
"A resilient community predicts and anticipates disasters; absorbs, responds, and recovers from the shock; and improvises and innovates in response to disasters."	Maguire and Hagan (2007)	Adaptation
"'Social resilience' is the capacity of a social entity (e.g., group or community) to 'bounce back' or respond positively to adversity."	Maguire and Hagan (2007)	Adaptation
"A positive trajectory of adaptation after a disturbance, stress, or adversity"	Norris and Stevens (2007)	Adaptation
"A process linking a network of adaptive capacities (resources with dynamic attributes) to adaptation after a disturbance or adversity"	Norris et al. (2008)	Adaptation
"The process through which mediating structures (schools, peer groups, family) and activity settings moderate the impact of oppressive systems"	Norris et al. (2008)	Adaptation
"The capability to bounce back and to use physical and economic resources effectively to aid recovery following exposure to hazards"	Norris et al. (2008)	Adaptation
"The ability of individuals and communities to deal with a state of continuous, long term stress"	Norris et al. (2008)	Adaptation
"The ability to find unknown inner strengths and resources in order to cope effectively"	Norris et al. (2008)	Basic
"The measure of adaptation and flexibility"	Norris et al. (2008)	Basic

Table A.2—Continued

Definition	Source	Basic/ Adaptation/ Growth
"The development of material, physical, socio-political, socio-cultural, and psychological resources that promote safety of residents and buffer adversity"	Norris et al. (2008)	Adaptation
"Individuals' sense of the ability of their own community to deal successfully with . . . ongoing political violence"	Norris et al. (2008)	Adaptation
"A community's capacities, skills, and knowledge that allow it to participate fully in recovery from disasters"	Norris et al. (2008)	Adaptation
"The ability of community members to take meaningful, deliberate, collective action to remedy the impact of a problem, including the ability to interpret the environment, intervene, and move on"	Norris et al. (2008)	Adaptation
"A process linking a network of adaptive capacities to a positive trajectory of functioning and adaptation after a disturbance"	Norris et al. (2008)	Adaptation
"The capacity for social units to mitigate the effects of hazards and to implement recovery activities in ways that limit social disruption and the effects of future events"	Pfefferbaum et al. (2008)	Adaptation
"A process evident in adaptation to threat or attack, stress, disruption, and security concerns"	Pfefferbaum et al. (2008)	Adaptation

Full Database of Resilience Literature

#1 Courtois, C.A., "Complex Trauma, Complex Reactions," *Psychological Trauma: Theory, Research, Practice, and Policy*, 2008. S(1): pp. 86–100.

#2 Gelkopf, M., et al., "The Impact of 'Training the Trainers' Course for Helping Tsunami-Survivor Children on Sri Lankan Disaster Volunteer Workers," *International Journal of Stress Management*, 2008. 15(2): pp. 117–135.

#3 Vernberg, E.M., et al., "Innovations in Disaster Mental Health: Psychological First Aid," *Professional Psychology: Research and Practice*, 2008. 39(4): pp. 381–388.

#5 Litz, B.T., and K. Salters-Pedneault, "Training Psychologists to Assess, Manage, and Treat Posttraumatic Stress Disorder: An Examination of the National Center for PTSD Behavioral Science Division Training Program," *Training and Education in Professional Psychology*, 2008. 2(2): pp. 67–74.

#6 Van Vliet, K.J., "Shame and Resilience in Adulthood: A Grounded Theory Study," *Journal of Counseling Psychology*, 2008. 55(2): pp. 233–245.

#7 Darwin, J.L., and K.I. Reich, "Reaching Out to the Families of Those Who Serve: The SOFAR Project," *Professional Psychology: Research and Practice*, 2006. 37(5): pp. 481–484.

#8 Creamer, M., and D. Forbes, "Treatment of Posttraumatic Stress Disorder in Military and Veteran Populations," *Psychotherapy: Theory, Research, Practice, Training*, 2004. 41(4): pp. 388–398.

#9 Agaibi, C.E. and J.P. Wilson, "Trauma, PTSD, and Resilience: A Review of the Literature," *Trauma Violence and Abuse*, 2005. 6(3): pp. 195–216.

#11 Ahmed, A.S., "Post-Traumatic Stress Disorder, Resilience and Vulnerability," *Advances in Psychiatric Treatment*, 2007. 13(5): pp. 369–375.

#17 Bartone, P.T. "The Need for Positive Meaning in Military Operations: Reflections on Abu Ghraib," in *112th Annual Convention of the American-Psychological-Association*. 2004. Honolulu, HI: Lawrence Erlbaum Assoc Inc.

#20 Benedek, D.M., and E.C. Ritchie, "'Just-in-Time' Mental Health Training and Surveillance for the Project HOPE Mission," *Mil Med*, 2006. 171(10 Suppl 1): pp. 63–65.

#21 Bonanno, G.A., "Loss, Trauma, and Human Resilience—Have We Underestimated the Human Capacity to Thrive After Extremely Aversive Events?" *American Psychologist*, 2004. 59(1): pp. 20–28.

#22 Bonanno, G.A., et al., "Psychological Resilience After Disaster—New York City in the Aftermath of the September 11th Terrorist Attack," *Psychological Science*, 2006. 17(3): pp. 181–186.

#23 Bonanno, G.A., et al., "What Predicts Psychological Resilience After Disaster? The Role of Demographics, Resources, and Life Stress," *Journal of Consulting and Clinical Psychology*, 2007. 75(5): pp. 671–682.

#24 Bonanno, G.A., C. Rennicke, and S. Dekel, "Self-Enhancement Among High-Exposure Survivors of the September 11th Terrorist Attack: Resilience or Social Maladjustment?" *Journal of Personality and Social Psychology*, 2005. 88(6): pp. 984–998.

#26 Bracha, H.S., "Human Brain Evolution and the 'Neuroevolutionary Time-Depth Principle': Implications for the Reclassification of Fear-Circuitry-Related Traits in DSM-V and for Studying Resilience to Warzone-Related Posttraumatic Stress Disorder," *Progress in Neuro-Psyhopharmacology and Biological Psychiatry*, 2006. 30: pp. 827–853.

#28 Bracha, H.S., et al. "Clinical Research Histomarkers for Objectively Estimating Premorbid Vagal Tone Chronology in Gulf War Veterans' Illnesses and in Acute Stress Reaction," in *Formal Descriptions of Developing Systems: Proceedings of the NATO Advanced Research Workshop*. 2003. National Center for PTSD, Department of Veterans Affairs, Spark M. Matsunaga VA Medical and Regional Office Center, Honolulu, Hawaii.

#30 Burnell, K.J., P.G. Coleman, and N. Hunt, "Falklands War Veterans' Perceptions of Social Support and the Reconciliation of Traumatic Memories," *Aging & Mental Health*, 2006. 10(3): pp. 282–289.

#31 Castro, C.A., and D. McGurk, "The Intensity of Combat and Behavioral Health Status," *Traumatology*, 2007. 13(4): pp. 6–23.

#33 Connor, K.M., "Assessment of Resilience in the Aftermath of Trauma," *Journal of Clinical Psychiatry*, 2006. 67(2): pp. 46–49.

#36 Decker, L.R., "Combat Trauma: Treatment from a Mystical/Spiritual Perspective," *Journal of Humanistic Psychology*, 2007. 47(30).

#38 Deuster, P.A., et al., "Human Performance Optimization: An Evolving Charge to the Department of Defense," *Military Medicine*, 2007. 172(11): p. 1133.

#41 Dohrenwend, B.P., et al., "Positive Tertiary Appraisals and Posttraumatic Stress Disorder in US Male Veterans of the War in Vietnam: The Roles of Positive Affirmation, Positive Reformulation, and Defensive Denial," *Journal of Consulting and Clinical Psychology*, 2004. 72(3): pp. 417–433.

#42 Dolan, C.A., and A.B. Adler, "Military Hardiness as a Buffer of Psychological Health on Return from Deployment," *Military Medicine*, 2006. 171(2): p. 93.

#43 Schiraldi, G.R., "World War II Survivors: Lessons in Resilience," *International Journal of Emergency Mental Health*, 2007. 9(1): pp. 47–53.

#45 Eid, J., and B.H. Johnsen, "Acute Stress Reactions After Submarine Accidents," *Mil Med*, 2002. 167(5): pp. 427–31.

#48 Fikretoglu, D., et al., "Validation of the Deployment Risk and Resilience Inventory in French-Canadian Veterans: Findings on the Relation Between Deployment Experiences and Postdeployment Health," *Canadian Journal of Psychiatry-Revue Canadienne De Psychiatrie*, 2006. 51(12): pp. 755–763.

#51 Friedman, M., and C. Higson-Smith, "Building Psychological Resilience: Learning from the South African Police Service," in *Promoting Capabilities to Manage Posttraumatic Stress: Perspectives on Resilience*, D. Paton, J.M. Violanti, and L.M. Smith, Editors. 2003, Charles C. Thomas: Springfield, Illinois. pp. 103–118.

#53 Frueh, C.B., et al., "US Department of Veterans Affairs Disability Policies for Posttraumatic Stress Disorder: Administrative Trends and Implications for Treatment, Rehabilitation, and Research," *American Journal of Public Health*, 2007. 97(12).

#54 Ghazinour, M. (2003). *Trauma and Resiliency: A Study of Refugees from Iran Resettled in Sweden*. Medical Dissertation. Department of Clinical Science, Umea University, Umea, Sweden.

55 Gold, P.B., et al., "Trauma Exposure, Resilience, Social Support, and PTSD Construct Validity Among Former Prisoners of War," *Social Psychiatry and Psychiatric Epidemiology*, 2000. 35(1): pp. 36–42.

57 Harris, D.A., "Dance/Movement Therapy Approaches to Fostering Resilience and Recovery Among African Adolescent Torture Survivors," *Torture*, 2007. 17(2): pp. 134–55.

59 Hart, C.L., *Posttraumatic Stress Symptomology in Aging Combat Veterans: The Direct and Buffering Effects of Stress and Social Support*, in Graduate School of Social Work. 2006, University of Pittsburgh: Pittsburgh, PA.

60 Hautamaki, A., and P.G. Coleman, "Explanation for Low Prevalence of PTSD Among Older Finnish War Veterans: Social Solidarity and Continued Significance Given to Wartime Sufferings," *Aging and Mental Health*, 2001. 5(2): pp. 165–174.

62 Hoge, E.A., E.D. Austin, and M.H. Pollack, "Resilience: Research Evidence and Conceptual Considerations for Posttraumatic Stress Disorder," *Depression and Anxiety*, 2007. 24(2): pp. 139–152.

65 Jennings, P.A., et al., "Combat Exposure, Perceived Benefits of Military Service, and Wisdom in Later Life—Findings from the Normative Aging Study," *Research on Aging*, 2006. 28(1): pp. 115–134.

66 Johnson, D.M., et al., "Emotional Numbing Weakens Abused Inner-City Women's Resiliency Resources," *Journal of Traumatic Stress*, 2007. 20(2): pp. 197–206.

67 Kimble, M., and M. Kaufman, "Clinical Correlates of Neurological Change in Posttraumatic Stress Disorder: An Overview of Critical Systems," *Psychiatric Clinics of North America*, 2004. 27: pp. 49–65.

68 King, L.A., et al., "Risk Factors for Mental, Physical, and Functional Health in Gulf War Veterans," *Journal of Rehabilitation Research and Development*, 2008. 45(3): pp. 395–408.

71 King, L.A., et al., "Deployment Risk and Resilience Inventory: A Collection of Measures for Studying Deployment-Related Experiences of Military Personnel and Veterans," *Military Psychology*, 2006. 18(2): pp. 89–120.

75 Larson, G.E., R.M. Highfill-McRoy, and S. Booth-Kewley, "Psychiatric Diagnoses in Historic and Contemporary Military Cohorts: Combat Deployment and the Healthy Warrior Effect," *American Journal of Epidemiology*, 2008. 167(11).

77 Lincoln, A., E. Swift, and M. Shorteno-Fraser, "Psychological Adjustment and Treatment of Children and Families with Parents Deployed in Military Combat," *Journal of Clinical Psychology*, 2008. 64(8): pp. 984–992.

78 Litz, B., "Has Resilience to Severe Trauma Been Underestimated?" *American Psychologist*, 2005. 60(3): p. 262.

79 Litz, B., "Research on the Impact of Military Trauma: Current Status and Future Directions," *Military Psychology*, 2007. 19(3): pp. 217–238.

81 Maguen, S., et al., "Description of Risk and Resilience Factors Among Military Medical Personnel Before Deployment to Iraq," *Mil Med*, 2008. 173(1): pp. 1–9.

82 Maguen, S., et al., "Posttraumatic Growth Among Gulf War I Veterans: The Predictive Role of Deployment-Related Experiences and Background Characteristics," *Journal of Loss and Trauma*, 2006. 11(5): pp. 373–388.

87 Morgan, C.A., et al., "Baseline Dissociation and Prospective Success in Special Forces Assessment and Selection," *Psychiatry*, 2008. July.

#91 Nemeroff, C.B., et al., "Posttraumatic Stress Disorder: A State-of-the-Science Review," *Journal of Psychiatric Research*, 2006. 40(1): pp. 1–21.

#93 Nitto, M.M., *An Investigation of Factors Contributing to Delays in the Onset of PTSD Among Vietnam Veterans*. 2001, University of Hartford. p. 93.

#95 Palmer, C., "A Theory of Risk and Resilience Factors in Military Families," *Military Psychology*, 2008. 20(3): pp. 205–217.

#97 Peach, H.G., "Further Support for the Families of Australia's War Veterans Requires a Broad Research Strategy," *MJA*, 2005. 183(3).

#98 Peres, J.F.P., et al., "Spirituality and Resilience in Trauma Victims," *Journal of Religion & Health*, 2007. 46(3): pp. 343–350.

#100 Punamaki, R.L., et al., "Psychological Distress and Resources Among Siblings and Parents Exposed to Traumatic Events," *International Journal of Behavioral Development*, 2006. 30(5): pp. 385–397.

#101 Qouta, S., et al., "Predictors of Psychological Distress and Positive Resources Among Palestinian Adolescents: Trauma, Child, and Mothering Characteristics," *Child Abuse and Neglect*, 2007. 31(7): pp. 699–717.

#102 Regel, S., "Post-Trauma Support in the Workplace: The Current Status and Practice of Critical Incident Stress Management (CISM) and Psychological Debriefing (PD) Within Organizations in the UK," *Occupational Medicine (Oxford, England)*, 2007. 57(6): pp. 411–416.

#105 Sammons, M.T., and S.V. Batten, "Psychological Services for Returning Veterans and Their Families: Evolving," *Journal of Clinical Psychology*, 2008. 64(8): pp. 921–927.

#107 Sharpley, J.G., et al., "Pre-Deployment Stress Briefing: Does It Have an Effect?" *Occupational Medicine*, 2008. 58(1): pp. 30–34.

#108 Smith, T.C., et al., "New Onset and Persistent Symptoms of Post-Traumatic Stress Disorder Self Reported After Deployment and Combat Exposures: Prospective Population Based US Military Cohort Study," *British Medical Journal*, 2008. 336(7639): pp. 366–376.

#109 Smith, T.C., et al., "Prior Assault and Posttraumatic Stress Disorder After Combat Deployment," *Epidemiology*, 2008. 19(3).

#113 Stetz, M.C., et al., "Psychiatric Diagnoses as a Cause of Medical Evacuation," *Aviation, Space, and Environmental Medicine*, 2005. 76(7).

#118 Tiet, Q.Q., et al., "Coping, Symptoms, and Functioning Outcomes of Patients with Posttraumatic Stress Disorder," *Journal of Traumatic Stress*, 2006. 19(6): pp. 799–811.

#120 Tucker, P.M., et al. "Physiologic Reactivity Despite Emotional Resilience Several Years After Direct Exposure to Terrorism," in *Groves Conference on Marriage and Family*, 2007. Oklahoma City, OK: American Psychiatric Publishing, Inc.

#122 Van Breda, A.D., "The Military Social Health Index: A Partial Multicultural Validation," *Military Medicine*, 2008. 173(5): pp. 480–487.

#123 Van Wijk, C.H., and A.H. Waters, "Positive Psychology Made Practical: A Case Study with Naval Specialists," *Military Medicine*, 2008. 173(5): p. 488.

#127 Waynick, T.C., et al., "Human Spirituality, Resilience, and the Role of Military Chaplains," in *Military Life: The Psychology of Serving in Peace and Combat*; Vol. 2: *Operational Stress*, A.B. Adler, C.A. Castro, and T.W. Britt, Editors. 2006, Praeger Security International: Westport, Connecticut. pp. 173–191.

#128 Waysman, M., J. Schwarzwald, and Z. Solomon, "Hardiness: An Examination of Its Relationship with Positive and Negative Long Term Changes Following Trauma," *Journal of Traumatic Stress*, 2001. 14(3).

#129 Wessely, S., "Risk, Psychiatry and the Military," *British Journal of Psychiatry*, 2005. 186: pp. 459–466.

#135 Zakin, G., Z. Solomon, and Y. Neria, "Hardiness, Attachment Style, and Long Term Psychological Distress Among Israeli POWs and Combat Veterans," *Personality and Individual Differences*, 2003. 34: pp. 819–829.

#136 Angelopoulos, P.A., et al., *Canadian Forces Training and Mental Preparation for Adversity: Empirical Review of Stoltz "Adversity Quotient (AQ) Training for Optimal Response to Adversity," A Review of the AQ Literature and Supporting Studies.* 2002, Defense Research and Development: Toronto, Canada. p. 42.

#137 Castro, C.A., et al. "Leader Actions to Enhance Soldier Resiliency in Combat," in *Human Dimensions in Military Operations: Military Leaders' Strategies for Addressing Stress and Psychological Support.* 2006. Neuilly-sur-France.

#140 Sharpe, G.E., and A. English, *Observations on the Association between Operational Readiness and Personal Readiness in the Canadian Forces.* 2006, Defence R&D Canada: Toronto, Canada.

#141 Huffman, A.H., A.B. Adler, and C.A. Castro, *The Impact of Deployment History on the Wellbeing of Military Personnel: The Gender Effect.* 2000, Army Medical Research Unit—Europe. p. 18.

#142 Laraway, L.A., *Stigma: "What Is It and Why Does the Operational Commander Need to Be Concerned?"* 2007, Naval War College, Joint Military Operations Department: Newport, RI. p. 26.

#143 Polusny, M.A., et al., *Longitudinal Risk and Resilience Factors Predicting Psychiatric Disruption, Mental Health Service Utilization & Military Retention in OIF National Guard Troops.* 2008, Minnesota University, Minneapolis: Minneapolis, MN. p. 38.

#144 Thompson, M.M., and M.A. Gignac, *A Model of Psychological Adaptation in Peace Support Operations: An Overview.* 2001, Defence and Civil Institute of Environmental Medicine: Downsview, Ontario—Canada. p. 50.

#145 Thompson, M.M., and D.R. McCreary, *Enhancing Mental Readiness in Military Personnel.* 2006, Defence Research and Development: Toronto, Canada. p. 13.

#148 Brailey, K., et al., "PTSD Symptoms, Life Events, and Unit Cohesion in U.S. Soldiers: Baseline Findings from the Neurocognition Deployment Health Study," *Journal of Traumatic Stress*, 2007. 20(4): pp. 495–503.

#149 Wald, J., et al., *Literature Review of Concepts: Psychological Resiliency.* 2006, British Columbia University: Vancouver, Canada. p. 134.

#152 Black, K., and M. Lobo, "A Conceptual Review of Family Resilience Factors," *Journal of Family Nursing*, 2008. 14(1): pp. 33–55.

#153 Boris, N.W., A.C. Ou, and R. Singh, "Preventing Post-Traumatic Stress Disorder After Mass Exposure to Violence," *Biosecurity and Bioterrorism*, 2005. 3(2): pp. 154–163.

#154 Marshall, K., *Bridging the Resilience Gap: Research to Practice.* 2001, University of Minnesota, National Resilience Resource Center: Minneapolis, MN.

#155 Earvolino-Ramirez, M., "Resilience: A Concept Analysis," *Nursing Forum*, 2007. 42(2): pp. 73–82.

#156 Fredrickson, B.L., et al., "What Good Are Positive Emotions in Crises? A Prospective Study of Resilience and Emotions Following the Terrorist Attacks on the United States on September 11th, 2001," *Journal of Personality and Social Psychology*, 2003. 84(2): pp. 365–376.

#159 MacDermid, S.M., et al., *Understanding and Promoting Resilience in Military Families*. 2008, Military Family Research Institute at Purdue Univeristy: West Lafayette.

#164 Walsh, F., "Family Resilience: A Framework for Clinical Practice," *Family Process*, 2003. 42(1).

#165 Walsh, F., "Traumatic Loss and Major Disasters: Strengthening Family and Community Resilience," *Family Process*, 2007. 46(2): pp. 207–227.

#166 Watson, P. J., E. C. Ritchie, et al., "Improving Resilience Trajectories Following Mass Violence and Disaster," in Ritchie, B.S., P.J. Watson, and M.J. Friedman, eds., *Interventions Following Mass Violence and Disasters: Strategies for Mental Health Practice*, New York: Guilford Press, 2006.

#169 Nucifora, F., et al., *Building Resistance, Resilience, and Recovery in the Wake of School and Workplace Violence*. 2007, Department of Psychiatry and Behavioral Health Sciences, Johns Hopkins University School of Medicine.

#171 Dirkzwager, A.J.E., et al., "Secondary Traumatization in Partners and Parents of Dutch Peacekeeping Soldiers," *Journal of Family Psychology*, 2005. 19(2): pp. 217–226.

#172 King, D.W., D.S. Vogt, and L.A. King, "Risk and Resilience Factors in the Etiology of Chronic Posttraumatic Stress Disorder," in *Early Intervention for Trauma and Traumatic Loss*, B. Litz, Editor. 2004, Guilford Press: New York, NY.

#174 Bartone, P.T., "Resilience Under Military Operational Stress: Can Leaders Influence Hardiness?" *Military Psychology*, 2006. 18(3 supp 1): pp. 131–148.

#175 Mancini, A.D., and G.A. Bonanno, "Resilience in the Face of Potential Trauma: Clinical Practices and Illustrations," *Journal of Clinical Psychology*, 2006. 62(8): pp. 971–985.

#176 Bonanno, G.A., et al., "The Importance of Being Flexible," *Psychological Science*, 2004. 15(7): pp. 482–487.

#177 Laffaye, C., et al., "Relationships Among PTSD Symptoms, Social Support, and Support Source in Veterans with Chronic PTSD," *Journal of Traumatic Stress*, 2008. 21(4): pp. 394–401.

#178 Conger, R.D., and K.J. Conger, "Resilience in Midwestern Families: Selected Findings from the First Decade of a Prospective, Longitudinal Study," *Journal of Marriage and Family*, 2002. 64(2): pp. 361–373.

#179 Botvin, G.J., and K.W. Griffin, "Life Skills Training: Empirical Findings and Future Directions," *Journal of Primary Prevention*, 2004. 25(2): pp. 211–232.

#180 Fergus, S., and M.A. Zimmerman, "Adolescent Resilience: A Framework for Understanding Healthy Development in the Face of Risk," *Annual Review of Public Health*, 2005. 26(1): pp. 399–419.

#181 Gibbs, D.A., S.L. Martin, and L.L. Kupper, "Child Maltreatment in Enlisted Soldiers' Families During Combat-Related Deployments," *Journal of the American Medical Association*, 2007. 298(5): pp. 528–535.

#182 Serido, J., D.M. Almeida, and E. Wethington, "Chronic Stressors and Daily Hassles: Unique and Interactive Relationships with Psychological Distress," *Journal of Health and Social Behavior*, 2004. 45(1): pp. 17–33.

#183 Tedeschi, R.G., and R.P. Kilmer, "Assessing Strengths, Resilience, and Growth to Guide Clinical Interventions" *Professional Psychology: Research and Practice*, 2005. 36(3): pp. 230–237.

184 Cozza, S.J., R.S. Chun, and J.A. Polo, "Military Families and Children During Operation Iraqi Freedom," *Psychiatric Quarterly*, 2005. 76(4): pp. 371–378.

185 Allison, S., et al., "What the Family Brings: Gathering Evidence for Strengths-Based Work," *Journal of Family Therapy*, 2003. 25(3): pp. 263–284.

186 Feeley, N., and L.N. Gottlieb, "Nursing Approaches for Working with Family Strengths and Resources," *Journal of Family Nursing*, 2000. 6(1): pp. 9–24.

187 Letourneau, N., et al., "Supporting Parents: Can Intervention Improve Parent-Child Relationships?" *Journal of Family Nursing*, 2001. 7(2): pp. 159–187.

188 Coleman, M., and L. Ganong, "Resilience and Families," *Family Relations*, 2002. 51(2): pp. 101–102.

189 Hipke, K.N., et al., "Predictors of Children's Intervention-Induced Resilience in a Parenting Program for Divorced Mothers," *Family Relations*, 2002. 51(2): pp. 121–129.

190 Middlemiss, W., "Prevention and Intervention: Using Resiliency-Based Multi-Setting Approaches and a Process-Orientation," *Child and Adolescent Social Work Journal*, 2005. 22(1): pp. 85–103.

191 Beardslee, W.R., "Resilience in Action," in *Out of the Darkened Room: When a Parent Is Depressed: Protecting the Children and Strengthening the Family*, 2002, Little, Brown: Boston.

192 Chen, H., et al., "Brief Report: The Emotional Distress in a Community After the Terrorist Attack on the World Trade Center," *Community Mental Health Journal*, 2003. 39(2): pp. 157–165.

193 Lester, P., *Project Focus: Families OverComing Under Stress*. 2008, University of California Los Angeles, National Child Traumatic Stress Network.

194 Harris, D.M., and J.T. Edwards, *A Preliminary Review of the OSCAR Pilot Program*. 2006, Center for Naval Analyses: Alexandra, VA.

195 Aisenberg, E., and T. Herrenkohl, "Community Violence in Context: Risk and Resilience in Children and Families," *Journal of Interpersonal Violence*, 2008. 23(3): pp. 296–315.

196 Patterson, J.M., "Integrating Family Resilience and Family Stress Therapy," *Journal of Marriage and Family*, 2002. 64(May 2002): pp. 349–360.

197 Barbarin, O.A., L. Richter, and T. deWet, "Exposure to Violence, Coping Resources, and Psychological Adjustment of South African Children," *American Journal of Orthopsychiatry*, 2001. 71(1).

198 Utku, F., and K. Chicinski, "Predicting Mental Illness in Soldiers: Pre-Deployment Screening for Vulnerability to Post-Traumatic Stress Disorder," *British Medical Journal*, 2006. 333(7578): p. 1123.

199 Thompson, M.M., and L. Pasto, "Psychological Interventions in Peace Support Operations: Current Practices and Future Challenges," in *The Psychology of the Peacekeeper: Lessons from the Field*, T. Britt and A.B. Adler, Editors. 2003, Praeger Publishers: Westport, CT.

201 Ano, G.G., and E.B. Vasconcelles, "Religious Coping and Psychological Adjustment to Stress: A Meta-Analysis," *Journal of Clinical Psychology*, 2005. 61(4): pp. 461–480.

203 Erbes, C.R., et al., "Couple Therapy with Combat Veterans and Their Partners," *Journal of Clinical Psychology: In Session*, 2008. 64(8): pp. 972–983.

204 Eaton, K.M., et al., "Prevalence of Mental Health Problems, Treatment Need, and Barriers to Care Among Primary Care-Seeking Spouses of Military Service Members Involved in Iraq and Afghanistan Deployments," *Military Medicine*, 2008. 173(11): p. 1051.

#205 McKeever, V.M., and M.E. Huff, "A Diathesis-Stress Model of Posttraumatic Stress Disorder: Ecological, Biological, and Residual Stress Pathways," *Review of General Psychology*, 2003. 7(3): pp. 237–250.

#206 Fraley, R.C., et al., "Attachment and Psychological Adaptation in High Exposure Survivors of the September 11th Attack on the World Trade Center," *Personality and Social Psychology Bulletin*, 2006. 32(4): pp. 538–551.

#207 Monson, C.M., S.J. Fredman, and K.C. Adair, "Cognitive-Behavioral Cojoint Therapy for Posttraumatic Stress Disorder: Application to Operation Enduring and Iraqi Freedom Veterans," *Journal of Clinical Psychology: In Session*, 2008. 64(8): pp. 958–971.

#208 Reger, G.M. and G.A. Gahm, "Virtual Reality Exposure Therapy for Active Duty Soldiers," *Journal of Clinical Psychology: In Session*, 2008. 64(8): pp. 940–946.

#209 Scarpa, A., S.C. Haden, and J. Hurley, "Community Violence Victimization and Symptoms of Posttraumatic Stress Disorder: The Moderating Effects of Coping and Social Support," *Journal of Interpersonal Violence*, 2006. 21: pp. 446–469.

#210 Shaw, A., S. Joseph, and A.P. Linley, "Religion, Spirituality, and Posttraumatic Growth: A Systematic Review," *Mental Health, Religion, and Culture*, 2005. 8(1): pp. 1–11.

#211 Silver, S.M., S. Rogers, and M. Russell, "Eye Movement Desensitization and Reprocessing (EMDR) in the Treatment of War Veterans," *Journal of Clinical Psychology: In Session*, 2008. 64(8): pp. 947–957.

#212 Condly, S.J., "Resilience in Children: A Review of Literature with Implications for Education," *Urban Education*, 2006. 41: pp. 211–236.

#213 Connor, K.M., and J.R.T. Davidson, "Development of a New Resilience Scale: The Connor-Davidson Resilience Scale (CD-RISC)," *Depression and Anxiety*, 2003. 18: pp. 76–82.

#214 Eriksson, M., and B. Lindstrom, "Antonovsky's Sense of Coherence Scale and the Relation with Health: A Systematic Review," *J Epidemiol Community Health*, 2006. 60: pp. 376–381.

#215 Everly, G.S., and J.T. Mitchell, "The Debriefing 'Controversy' and Crisis Intervention: A Review of Lexical and Substantive Issues," *International Journal of Emergency Mental Health*, 2000. 2(4): pp. 211–225.

#216 Fredrickson, B.L., "The Role of Positive Emotions in Positive Psychology: The Broaden-and-Build Theory of Positive Emotions," *American Psychologist*, 2001. 56(3): pp. 218–226.

#217 Greenberg, N., V. Langston, and N. Jones, "Trauma Risk Management: (TRiM) in the UK Armed Forces," *JR Army Med Corps*, 2008. 154(2): pp. 123–126.

#218 Paton, D., "Critical Incident Stress Risk in Police Officers: Managing Resilience and Vulnerability," *Traumatology*, 2006. 12(198): pp. 198–205.

#219 Jarrett, T.A., "Warrior Resilience Training in Operation Iraqi Freedom: Combining Rational Emotive Behavior Therapy, Resiliency, and Positive Psychology," *Army Medical Department Journal*, 2008 (July–September 2008).

#221 Carver, C.S., "Resilience and Thriving: Issues, Models, and Linkages," *Journal of Social Issues*, 1998. 54(2): pp. 245–266.

#222 Sharkansky, E.J., et al., "Coping with Gulf War Combat Stress: Mediating and Moderating Effects," *Journal of Abnormal Psychology*, 2000. 109(2): pp. 188–197.

#223 Barton, W., "Methodological Challenges in the Study of Resilience," in *Handbook for Working with Children and Youth: Pathways to Resilience Across Cultures and Contexts*, M. Ungar, Editor. 2003. Sage Publications: Thousand Oaks, CA, pp. 135–147.

#224 Ungar, M., and E. Terem, "Qualitative Resilience Research," in *Handbook for Working with Children and Youth: Pathways to Resilience Across Cultures and Contexts*, M. Ungar, Editor. 2003, Sage Publications: Thousand Oaks, CA, pp. 149–163.

#225 Faber, A.J., et al., "Ambiguous Absence, Ambiguous Presence: A Qualitative Study of Military Reserve Families in Wartime," *Journal of Family Psychology*, 2008. 22(2): pp. 222–230.

#226 Hoge, C.W., et al., "Combat Duty in Iraq and Afghanistan, Mental Health Problems, and Barriers to Care," *New England Journal of Medicine*, 2004. 351(1): pp. 13–22.

#227 Huebner, A.J., and J.A. Mancini, *Adjustments Among Adolescents in Military Families When a Parent Is Deployed*. 2005, Military Family Research Institute at Purdue University.

#228 Luthar, S.S., and D. Cicchetti, "The Construct of Resilience: Implications for Interventions and Social Policies," *Developmental Psychopathology*, 2000. 12(4): pp. 857–885.

#229 Tusaie, K., and J. Dyer, "Resilience: A Historical Review of the Construct," *Holist Nurs Pract*, 2004. 18(1): pp. 3–8.

#230 Wiens, T.W., and P. Boss, "Maintaining Family Resiliency Before, During, and After Military Separation," in *Military Life: The Psychology of Serving in Peace and Combat*, T.W. Britt, A.B. Adler, and C.A. Castro, Editors. 2006, Praeger Security International: Westport, Connecticut.

#231 Alriksson-Schmidt, A.I., J. Wallander, and F. Biasini, "Quality of Life and Resilience in Adolescents with a Mobility Disability," *Journal of Pediatric Psychology*, 2007. 32(3): pp. 1–10.

#232 Bolton, E.E., et al., "The Impact of Homecoming Reception on the Adaptation of Peacekeepers Following Deployment," *Military Psychology*, 2002. 14(3): pp. 241–251.

#233 Calhoun, L.G., and R.G. Tedeschi, "The Foundations of Posttraumatic Growth: New Considerations," *Psychological Inquiry*, 2004. 15(1): pp. 93–102.

#234 Charney, D.S., "Psychobiological Mechanisms of Resilience and Vulnerability: Implications for Successful Adaptation to Extreme Stress," *American Journal of Psychiatry*, 2004. 161(February): pp. 195–216.

#236 Luthar, S.S., D. Cicchetti, and B. Becker, "The Construct of Resilience: Implications for Interventions and Social Policies," *Child Development*, 2000. 71(3): pp. 543–562.

#237 Ness, G., and N. Macaskill, "Preventing PTSD: The Value of Inner Resourcefulness and a Sense of Personal Control of a Situation: Is it a Matter of Problem-Solving or Anxiety Management?" *Behavioural and Cognitive Psychotherapy*, 2003. 31: pp. 463–466.

#238 Bonanno, G.A., and A.D. Mancini, "The Human Capacity to Thrive in the Face of Potential Trauma," *Pediatrics*, 2008. 121: pp. 369–375.

#239 Novaco, R.W., T.M. Cook, and I.G. Sarason, "Military Recruit Training: An Arena for Stress-Coping Skills," in *Stress Reduction and Prevention*, D. Meichenbaum and M.E. Jaremko, Editors. 1983, Plenum Press: New York, NY. p. 3.

#240 Van Breda, A.D., *Resilience Theory: A Literature Review*. 2001, South African Military Health Service, Military Psychological Institute, Social Work Research & Development: Pretoria, South Africa.

#241 Norris, F.H., and S.P. Stevens, "Community Resilience and the Principles of Mass Trauma Intervention," *Psychiatry*, 2007. 70(4): pp. 320–328.

#242 Gurwitch, R.H., et al., *Building Community Resilience for Children and Families*. 2007, Terrorism and Disaster Center at the University of Oklahoma Health Sciences Center, National Child Traumatic Stress Network: Oklahoma City. p. 74.

#243 O'Donnell, D.A., M.E. Schwab-Stone, and A.Z. Muyeed, "Multidimensional Resilience in Urban Children Exposed to Community Violence," *Child Development*, 2002. 73(4): pp. 1265–1282.

#244 Pfefferbaum, R.L., et al., "Factors in the Development of Community Resilience to Disasters," in *Intervention and Resilience After Mass Trauma*, M. Blumenfield and R.J. Ursano, Editors. 2008, Cambridge University Press: Cambridge, UK.

#245 Hobfoll, S.E., et al., "Five Essential Elements of Immediate and Mid-Term Mass Trauma Intervention: Empirical Evidence," *Psychiatry*, 2007. 70(4): pp. 283–315.

#246 Masten, A.S., "Ordinary Magic: Resilience Processes in Development," *American Psychologist*, 2001. 56(3): pp. 227–238.

#247 Bliese, P.D., et al., "Timing of Postcombat Mental Health Assessments," *Psychological Services*, 2007. 4(3): pp. 141–148.

#248 Conger, R.D., M.A. Rueter, and G.H.J. Elder, "Couple Resilience to Economic Pressure," *Journal of Personality and Social Psychology*, 1999. 76(1): pp. 54–71.

#249 Jensen, J.M., and M.W. Fraser, "A Risk and Resilience Framework for Child, Youth, and Family Policy," in *Social Policy for Children and Families: A Risk and Resilience Perspective*, J.M. Jensen and M.W. Fraser, Editors. 2005, Sage Publications: Thousand Oaks, CA.

#250 Vogt, D.S., and L.R. Tanner, "Risk and Resilience Factors for Posttraumatic Stress Symptomatology in Gulf War I Veterans," *Journal of Traumatic Stress*, 2007. 20(1): pp. 27–38.

#251 King, D.W., et al., "Directionality of the Association Between Social Support and Posttraumatic Stress Disorder: A Longitudinal Investigation," *Journal of Applied Social Psychology*, 2006. 36(12): pp. 2980–2992.

#252 Maguire, B., and P. Hagan, "Disasters and Communities: Understanding Social Resilience," *Australian Journal of Emergency Management*, 2007. 22(2): pp. 16–20.

#253 Speckhard, A., "Innoculating Resilience to Terrorism: Acute and Posttraumatic Stress Responses in U.S. Military, Foreign, and Civilian Services Serving Overseas After September 11th," *Traumatology*, 2002. 8(June): pp. 103–130.

#254 Haglund, M.E.M., et al., "Psychobiological Mechanisms of Resilience: Relevance to Prevention and Treatment of Stress-Related Psychopathology," *Development and Psychopathology*, 2007. 19: pp. 889–920.

#255 Tedeschi, R.G., and L.G. Calhoun, "Posttraumatic Growth: Conceptual Foundations and Empirical Evidence," *Psychological Inquiry*, 2004. 15(1): pp. 1–15.

#256 Bliese, P.D., et al., "Validating the Primary Care Posttraumatic Stress Disorder Screen and the Posttraumatic Stress Disorder Checklist with Soldiers Returning from Combat," *Journal of Consulting and Clinical Psychology*, 2008. 76(2): pp. 272–281.

#257 King, L.A., et al., "Resilience-Recovery Factors in Post-Traumatic Stress Disorder Among Female and Male Vietnam Veterans: Hardiness, Postwar Social Support, and Additional Stressful Life Events," *Journal of Personality and Social Psychology*, 1998. 74(2): pp. 420–434.

#258 Bracha, H.S., and J.O. Bienvenu, "Rapidly Assessing Trauma Exposure and Stress Resilience Following Large-Scale Disasters," *Journal of Emergency Management*, 2005. 3(6): pp. 27–31.

#259 Meichenbaum, D., and R. Cameron, "Stress Inoculation Training: Toward a General Paradigm for Training Coping Skills," in *Stress Reduction and Prevention*, D. Meichenbaum and M.E. Jaremko, Editors. 1983, Plenum Press: New York, NY.

#260 King, D.W., et al., "Posttraumatic Stress Disorder in a National Sample of Female and Male Vietnam Veterans: Risk Factors, War Zone Stressors, and Resilience-Recovery Variables," *Journal of Abnormal Psychology*, 1999. 108(1): pp. 164–170.

#261 Dekel, R., and H. Goldblott, "Is There Intergenerational Transmission of Trauma? The Case of Combat Veterans' Children," *American Journal of Orthopsychiatry*, 2008. 78(3): pp. 281–289.

#262 Miller, M.W., "Personality and the Etiology and Expression of PTSD: A Three-Factor Model Perspective," *Clinical Psychology: Science and Practice*, 2003. 10(4): pp. 373–393.

#263 Hjemdal, O., et al., "Predicting Psychiatric Symptoms," *Clinical Psychology and Psychotherapy*, 2006. 13: pp. 194–201.

#265 Maeseele, P.A., et al., "Psychosocial Resilience in the Face of a Mediated Terrorist Event," *Media, War, and Conflict*, 2008. 1(1): pp. 50–69.

#267 Rutter, M., "Resilience Concepts and Findings: Implications for Family Therapy," *Journal of Family Therapy*, 1999. 21: pp. 119–144.

#268 Bliese, P.D., and C.A. Castro, "The Soldier Adaptation Model (SAM): Applications to Peacekeeping Research," in *The Psychology of the Peacekeeper: Lessons from the Field*, T. Britt and A.B. Adler, Editors. 2003, Praeger: Westport, Connecticut.

#269 Garb, H.N., and J. Cigrang, "Psychological Screening: Predicting Resilience to Stress," in *Biobehavioral Resilience to Stress*, B.J. Lukey and V. Tepe, Editors. 2008, CRC Press: Boca Raton, FL.

#270 Ritchie, E.C., et al., "Resilience and Military Psychology," in *Biobehavioral Resilience to Stress*, B.J. Lukey and V. Tepe, Editors. 2008, CRC Press: Boca Raton, FL.

#271 Campbell, D., K. Campbell, and J. Ness, "Resilience Through Leadership," in *Biobehavioral Resilience to Stress*, B.J. Lukey and V. Tepe, Editors. 2008, CRC Press: Boca Raton, FL.

#272 Southwick, S., et al., "Adaptation to Stress and Psychobiological Mechanisms of Resilience," in *Biobehavioral Resilience to Stress*, B.J. Lukey and V. Tepe, Editors. 2008, CRC Press: Boca Raton, FL.

#273 Friedl, K., and D. Penetar, "Resilience and Survival in Extreme Environments," in *Biobehavioral Resilience to Stress*, B.J. Lukey and V. Tepe, Editors. 2008, CRC Press: Boca Raton, FL.

#274 Staal, M., et al., "Cognitive Performance and Resilience to Stress," in *Biobehavioral Resilience to Stress*, B.J. Lukey and V. Tepe, Editors. 2008, CRC Press: Boca Raton, FL.

#275 Rohall, D., and J. Martin, "The Impact of Social Structural Conditions on Psychological Resilience to Stress," in *Biobehavioral Resilience to Stress*, B.J. Lukey and V. Tepe, Editors. 2008, CRC Press: Boca Raton, FL.

#276 Tepe, V., and J. Lukey, "Resilience: Toward the State of the Possible," in *Biobehavioral Resilience to Stress*, B.J. Lukey and V. Tepe, Editors. 2008, CRC Press: Boca Raton, FL.

#277 Tugade, M.M., and B.L. Fredrickson, "Resilient Individuals Use Positive Emotions to Bounce Back from Negative Emotional Experiences," *Journal of Personality and Social Psychology*, 2004. 86(2): pp. 320–333.

#278 Pfefferbaum, B., et al., "Building Resilience to Mass Trauma Events," in *Handbook on Injury and Violence Prevention*, L.S. Doll, et al., Editors. 2007, Centers for Disease Control and Prevention, National Center for Injury Prevention and Control: Atlanta, GA.

#279 Calhoun, L.G., and R.G. Tedeschi, "The Foundations of Posttraumatic Growth: An Expanded Framework," in *Handbook of Posttraumatic Growth: Research and Practice*, L.G. Calhoun and R.G. Tedeschi, Editors. 2006, Lawrence Erlbaum Associates: Mahwah, NJ.

#280 Lepore, S., and T. Revenson, "Relationships Between Posttraumatic Growth and Resilience: Recovery, Resistance, and Reconfiguration," in *Handbook of Posttraumatic Growth: Research and Practice*, L.G. Calhoun and R.G. Tedeschi, Editors. 2006, Lawrence Erlbaum Associates: Mahwah, NJ.

#281 Rosner, R., and S. Powell, "Posttraumatic Growth After War," in *Handbook of Posttraumatic Growth: Research and Practice*, L.G. Calhoun and R.G. Tedeschi, Editors. 2006, Lawrence Erlbaum Associates: Mahwah, NJ.

#282 Meichenbaum, D., "Posttraumatic Growth After War," in *Handbook of Posttraumatic Growth: Research and Practice*, L.G. Calhoun and R.G. Tedeschi, Editors. 2006, Lawrence Erlbaum Associates: Mahwah, NJ.

#283 Bliese, P.D., "Social Climates: Drivers of Soldier Well-Being and Resilience," in *Military Life*, C.A. Castro, A.B. Adler, and T. Britt, Editors. 2006, Greenwood Publishing Group: Santa Barbara, CA.

#284 Sinclair, R.R., and J.S. Tucker, "Stress-CARE: An Integrated Model of Individual Differences in Soldier Performance Under Stress," in *Military Life*, C.A. Castro, T. Britt, and A.B. Adler, Editors. 2006, Greenwood Publishing Group: Santa Barbara, CA.

#285 Litz, B., and M.J. Gray, "Early Intervention for Trauma in Adults," in *Early Intervention for Trauma and Traumatic Loss*, B. Litz, Editor. 2004, Guilford Press: New York, NY.

#286 Castro, C.A., C.C. Engel, and A.B. Adler, "The Challenge of Providing Mental Health Prevention and Early Intervention in the U.S. Military," in *Early Intervention for Trauma and Traumatic Loss*, B. Litz, Editor. 2004, New York, NY: Guilford Press.

#287 Tanyi, R.A., "Spirituality and Family Nursing: Spiritual Assessment and Interventions for Families," *Journal of Advanced Nursing*, 2006. 53(3): pp. 287–294.

#288 Taylor, S., "Adjustment to Threatening Events: A Theory of Cognitive Adaptation," *American Psychologist*, 1983(November): pp. 1161–1173.

#289 Hobfoll, S.E., et al., "War-Related Stress: Addressing the Stress of War and Other Traumatic Events," *American Psychologist*, 1991. 46(8): pp. 848–855.

#290 Schiraldi, G.R., and S.L. Brown, "Primary Prevention for Mental Health: Results of an Exploratory Cognitive-Behavioral College Course," *Journal of Primary Prevention*, 2001. 22(1): pp. 55–67.

#291 Keane, T.M., et al., "Social Support in Vietnam Veterans with Posttraumatic Stress Disorder: A Comparative Analysis," *Journal of Consulting and Clinical Psychology*, 1985. 53(1): pp. 95–102.

#292 Solomon, Z., M. Mikulincer, and E. Avitzur, "Coping, Locus of Control, Social Support, and Combat-Related Posttraumatic Stress Disorder: A Prospective Study," *Journal of Personality and Social Psychology*, 1988. 55(2): pp. 279–285.

#293 Affleck, G., and H. Tennen, "Construing Benefits from Adversity: Adaptational Significance and Dispositional Underpinnings," *Journal of Personality*, 1996. 64(4): pp. 899–922.

#294 Fredrickson, B.L., "Cultivating Positive Emotions to Optimize Health and Well-Being," *Prevention and Treatment*, 2000. 3(1).

#295 Butler, L.D., L.A. Morland, and G.A. Leskin, "Psychological Resilience in the Face of Terrorism," in *Psychology of Terrorism*, Bonger, et al., Editors. 2007, Oxford University Press: Oxford, UK.

#296 Adler, A.B., C.A. Castro, and D. McGurk, "Time-Driven Battlemind Psychological Debriefing: A Group-Level Early Intervention in Combat," *Military Medicine*, 2009. 174(1): pp. 21–28.

#297 Friesen, B.J., and E. Brennan, "Strengthening Families and Communities: System Building for Resilience," in *Handbook for Working with Children and Youth*, M. Ungar, Editor. 2005, Sage Publications: Thousand Oaks, CA.

#298 Boyden, J., and G. Mann, "Children's Risk, Resilience, and Coping in Extreme Situations," in *Handbook for Working with Children and Youth*, M. Ungar, Editor. 2005, Sage Publications: Thousand Oaks, CA.

#299 Schwerin, M.J., "Quality of Life and Subjective Well-Being Among Military Personnel: An Organizational Response to the Challenges of Military Life," in *Military Life*, C.A. Castro, A.B. Adler, and T. Britt, Editors. 2006, Greenwood Publishing Group: Santa Barbara, CA.

#300 Siebold, G.L., "Military Group Cohesion," in *Military Life*, T. Britt, C.A. Castro, and A.B. Adler, Editors. 2006, Greenwood Publishing Group: Santa Barbara, CA.

#301 Shalev, A.Y., and Y.L.E. Errera, "Resilience Is the Default: How Not to Miss It," in *Intervention and Resilience After Mass Trauma*, M. Blumenfield and R.J. Ursano, Editors. 2008, Cambridge University Press: Cambridge, UK.

#302 Watson, P.J., "Psychological First Aid," in *Intervention and Resilience After Mass Trauma*, ed. M. Blumenfield and R.J. Ursano. 2008, Cambridge, UK: Cambridge University Press.

#303 Ursano, R.J., and M. Blumenfield, "Epilogue," in *Intervention and Resilience After Mass Trauma*, M. Blumenfield and R.J. Ursano, Editors. 2008, Cambridge University Press: Cambridge, UK.

#304 Maddi, S.R., and D.M. Khoshaba, "Hardiness Training for Resiliency and Leadership," in *Promoting Capabilities to Manage Posttraumatic Stress*, D. Paton, J.M. Violanti, and L.M. Smith, Editors. 2003, Charles C. Thomas Publisher, Ltd.: Springfield, Illinois.

#305 Bartone, P.T., "Hardiness as a Resiliency Resource Under High Stress Conditions," in *Promoting Capabilities to Manage Posttraumatic Stress*, D. Paton, J.M. Violanti, and L.M. Smith, Editors. 2003, Charles C. Thomas Publisher, Ltd.: Springfield, Illinois.

#306 Bartone, P.T., et al., "Team Resilience," in *Promoting Capabilities to Manage Posttraumatic Stress*, D. Paton, J.M. Violanti, and L.M. Smith, Editors. 2003, Charles C. Thomas Publisher, Ltd.: Springfield, Illinois.

#307 Pollock, C., et al., "Training for Resilience," in *Promoting Capabilities to Manage Posttraumatic Stress*, D. Paton, J.M. Violanti, and L.M. Smith, Editors. 2003, Charles C. Thomas Publisher, Ltd.: Springfield, Illinois.

#308 Dunning, C., "Sense of Coherence in Managing Traumatic Workers," in *Promoting Capabilities to Manage Posttraumatic Stress*, D. Paton, J.M. Violanti, and L.M. Smith, Editors. 2003, Charles C. Thomas Publisher, Ltd.: Springfield, Illinois.

#309 Johnston, P., and D. Paton, "Environmental Resilience and Psychological Empowerment in High-Risk Professions," in *Promoting Capabilities to Manage Posttraumatic Stress*, D. Paton, J.M. Violanti, and L.M. Smith, Editors. 2003, Charles C. Thomas Publisher, Ltd.: Springfield, Illinois.

#310 Payne, R.L., and M. Clark, "The Process of Trusting: Its Relevance to Vulnerability and Resilience in Traumatic Situations," in *Promoting Capabilities to Manage Posttraumatic Stress*, D. Paton, J.M. Violanti, and L.M. Smith, Editors. 2003, Charles C. Thomas Publisher, Ltd.: Springfield, Illinois.

#311 Shakespeare-Finch, J., D. Paton, and J.M. Violanti, "The Family: Resilience Resource and Resilience Needs," in *Promoting Capabilities to Manage Posttraumatic Stress*, D. Paton, J.M. Violanti, and L.M. Smith, Editors. 2003, Charles C. Thomas Publisher, Ltd.: Springfield, Illinois.

#312 Smith, L.M., and J.M. Violanti, "Risk Response Model," in *Promoting Capabilities to Manage Posttraumatic Stress*, D. Paton, J.M. Violanti, and L.M. Smith, Editors. 2003, Charles C. Thomas Publisher, Ltd.: Springfield, Illinois.

#313 Paton, D., J.M. Violanti, and L.M. Smith, "Posttraumatic Psychological Stress: Individual, Group, and Organizational Perspectives on Resilience and Growth," in *Promoting Capabilities to Manage Posttraumatic Stress*, D. Paton, J.M. Violanti, and L.M. Smith, Editors. 2003, Charles C. Thomas Publisher, Ltd.: Springfield, Illinois.

#314 Yehuda, R., et al., "Developing an Agenda for Translational Studies of Resilience and Vulnerability Following Trauma Exposure," *New York Academy of Sciences*, 2006. 1071: pp. 379–396.

#315 Calhoun, L.G., and R.G. Tedeschi, "Routes to Posttraumatic Growth Through Cognitive Processing," in *Promoting Capabilities to Manage Posttraumatic Stress*, D. Paton, J.M. Violanti, and L.M. Smith, Editors. 2003, Charles C. Thomas Publisher, Ltd.: Springfield, Illinois.

#316 Norris, F.H., et al., "Community Resilience as a Metaphor, Theory, Set of Capacities, and Strategy for Disaster Readiness," *American Journal of Community Psychology*, 2008. 41: pp. 127–150.

#317 Bowen, G.L., et al., "Promoting the Adaptation of Military Families: An Empirical Test of a Community Practice Model," *Family Relations*, 2003. 52(1): pp. 33–44.

#318 Bell, C.C., "Cultivating Resiliency in Youth," *Journal of Adolescent Health*, 2001. 29: pp. 375–381.

#319 Rose, S.C., et al., *Psychological Debriefing for Preventing Post Traumatic Stress Disorder (PTSD) Review*, 2009, Cochrane Collaboration.

#320 Friborg, O., et al., "A New Rating Scale for Adult Resilience: What Are the Central Protective Resources Behind Health Adjustment," *International Journal of Methods in Psychiatric Research*, 2006 12(2): pp. 65–76.

#321 Gillham, J.E., et al., "School-Based Prevention of Depressive Symptoms: A Randomized Controlled Study of the Effectiveness and Specificity of the Penn Resilience Program," *Journal of Consulting and Clinical Psychology*, 2007. 75(1): pp. 9–19.

#322 Adler, A.B., et al., "International Military Leaders' Survey on Operational Stress," *Military Medicine*, 2008. 173(1): pp. 10–16.

#323 Stetz, M.C., et al., "Stress, Mental Health, and Cognition: A Brief Review of Relationships and Countermeasures," *Aviation, Space, and Environmental Medicine*, 2007. 78(5): pp. 252–260.

#324 Batzer, W.B., et al., "Cohesion, Burnout, and Past Trauma in Tri-Service Medical and Support Personnel," *Military Medicine*, 2007. 172(3): pp. 266–272.

#325 Maddi, S.R., "Relevance of Hardiness Assessment and Training to the Military Context," *Military Psychology*, 2007. 19(1): pp. 61–70.

#326 Morgan, C.A., et al., "Relation Between Cardiac Vagal Tone and Performance in Male Military Personnel Exposed to High Stress: Three Prospective Studies," *Psychophysiology*, 2007. 44: pp. 120–127.

#327 Meyerhoff, J.I., et al., "Evaluating Performance of Law Enforcement Personnel During a Stressful Training Scenario," *New York Academy of Sciences*, 2004. 1032: pp. 250–253.

#328 Harter, J.K., F.L. Schmidt, and T.L. Hayes, "Business-Unit-Level Relationship Between Employee Satisfaction, Employee Engagement, and Business Outcomes: A Meta-Analysis," *Journal of Applied Psychology*, 2002. 87(2): pp. 268–279.

#329 Zach, S., S. Raviv, and R. Inbar, "The Benefits of a Graduated Training Program for Security Officers on Physical Performance in Stressful Situations," *International Journal of Stress Management*, 2007. 14(4): pp. 350–369.

#330 Williams, A., et al., "Psychosocial Effects of the Boot Strap Intervention in Navy Recruits," *Military Medicine*, 2004. 169(10): pp. 814–820.

#331 Williams, A., et al., "STARS: Strategies to Assist Navy Recruits' Success," *Military Medicine*, 2007. 172(9): pp. 942–949.

#332 Gill, Jessica, et al., *Dispositional Traits and Social Factors Related to Trauma Resilience: Implications for Therapy*, unpublished manuscript, 2010.

#333 Bartone, P.T., T. Spinosa, and J. Robb. "Psychological Hardiness Is Related to Baseline High-Density Lipoprotein (HDL) Cholesterol Levels," in *Association for Psychological Science Convention*. 2009. San Francisco, CA.

#334 Loehr, J., and T. Schwartz, "The Making of a Corporate Athlete," *Harvard Business Review*, 2001. January pp. 120–126.

#335 Schwartz, T., and C. McCarthy, "Manage Your Energy, Not Your Time," *Harvard Business Review*, October 2007.

#336 Meichenbaum, D., "What Do Resilient Individuals Do: Implications for Psychotherapists," L. Meredith, Editor. 2009. E-Summits, Presentation Notes.

#337 Fry, L.W., "Toward a Theory of Spiritual Leadership," *Leadership Quarterly*, 2003. 14: pp. 693–727.

#338 Fry, L.W., "Spiritual Leadership: State-of-the-Art and Future Directions for Theory, Research, and Practice," in *Spirituality in Business: Theory, Practice, and Future Directions*, J. Biberman and L. Tishman, Editors. 2008, Palgrave Macmillan: New York, NY.

#340 Adler, A.B., et al., "Battlemind Debriefing and Battlemind Training as Early Interventions with Soldiers Returning from Iraq: Randomized by Platoon," *Journal of Consulting and Clinical Psychology*, 2009. 77(5): pp. 928–940.

#341 Litz, B., et al., "Moral Injury and Moral Repair in War Veterans: A Preliminary Model and Intervention Strategy," *Clinical Psychology Review*, 2009. 29: pp. 695–706.

#342 Faran, M.E., et al., "School-Based Mental Health on a United States Army Installation," in *Handbook of School Mental Health Advancing Practice and Research*, M.D. Weist, S.W. Evans, and N.A. Lever, Editors. 2002, Springer: New York, NY.

#343 Tiller, W.A., R. McCraty, and M. Atkinson, "Cardiac Coherence: A New, Noninvasive Measure of Autonomic Nervous System Order," *Alternative Therapies*, 1996. 2(1): pp. 52–65.

#344 Luskin, F., et al., "A Controlled Pilot Study of Stress Management Training of Elderly Patients with Congestive Heart Failure," *Preventive Cardiology*, 2002(Fall): pp. 168–176.

#345 McCraty, R., et al., "The Effects of Emotions on Short-Term Power Spectrum Analysis of Heart Rate Variability," *American Journal of Cardiology*, 1995. 76(4): pp. 1089–1093.

#346 McCraty, R., M. Atkinson, and D. Tomasino, "Impact of Workplace Stress Reduction Program on Blood Pressure and Emotional Health in Hypertensive Employees," *Journal of Alternative and Complementary Medicine*, 2003. 9(3): pp. 355–369.

#347 Rozman, D., et al., "A Pilot Intervention Program That Reduced Psychological Symptomatology in Individuals with Human Immunodeficiency Virus," *Complementary Therapies in Medicine*, 1996. 4: pp. 226–232.

#348 McCraty, R., et al., "The Impact of an Emotional Self-Management Skills Course on Psychosocial Functioning and Autonomic Recovery to Stress in Middle School Children," *Integrative Physiological and Behavioral Science*, 1999. 34(4): pp. 246–268.

#349 McCraty, R., "From Depletion to Renewal: Positive Emotions and Heart Rhythm Coherence Feedback," *Biofeedback*, 2008. 36(1): pp. 30–34.

#350 McCraty, R., et al., "The Impact of a New Emotional Self-Management Program on Stress, Emotions, Heart Rate Variability, DHEA and Cortisol," *Integrative Physiological and Behavioral Science*, 1998. 33(2): pp. 151–170.

#351 McCraty, R., et al., "Hew Hope for Correctional Officers: An Innovative Program for Reducin Stress and Health Risks," *Applied Psychophysiology and Biofeedback*, 2009. 34(4).

#352 Harter, J.K., and V.F. Gurley, "Measuring Well-Being in the United States," *Association for Psychological Science*, 2008. 21(8): pp. 23–26.

#353 Stanley, E.A., et al., "Mind Fitness in Counterinsurgency: Addressing the Cognitive Requirements of Population-Centric Operations," *Military Review*, 2010. 90(1).

#354 Stanley, E.A., "Neuroplasticity, Mind Fitness, and Military Effectiveness," in *The "New" Biological Warfare: Biotechnology and the Future of America's Military*, M. Drapeau, Editor. 2009, National Defense University Press: Washington, D.C.

#356 Stanley, E.A., and A.P. Jha, "Mind Fitness and Mental Armor: Enhancing Performance and Building Warrior Resilience," *Joint Force Quarterly*, 2009. 55(October): pp. 145–151.

#357 Gahm, G.A., et al., "History and Implementation of the Fort Lewis Soldier Wellness Assessment Program (SWAP)," *Military Medicine*, 2009. 174(7): pp. 721–727.

#358 Mancini, J.A., et al., "Preventing Intimate Partner Violence: A Community Capacity Approach," *Journal of Aggression, Maltreatment, & Trauma*, 2006. 13(3/4): pp. 203–227.

#359 Bowen, G.L., et al., "Community Capacity: Antecedents and Consequences," *Journal of Community Practice*, 2000. 8(2).

#360 Mancini, J.A., G.L. Bowen, and J.A. Martin, "Community Social Organization: A Conceptua Linchpin in Examining Families in the Context of Communities," *Family Relations*, 2005. 54(December): pp. 570–582.

#361 Bowen, G.L., J.A. Martin, and J.A. Mancini, *Communities in Blue for the 21st Century*. 1999, Caliber Associates: Fairfax, VA.

Database of Resilience Literature with Moderate or Strong Evidence by Factor

Individual-Level Factors

Coping

#2 Gelkopf, M., et al., "The Impact of 'Training the Trainers' Course for Helping Tsunami-Survivor Children on Sri Lankan Disaster Volunteer Workers," *International Journal of Stress Management*, 2008. 15(2): pp. 117–135.

#3 Vernberg, E.M., et al., "Innovations in Disaster Mental Health: Psychological First Aid," *Professional Psychology: Research and Practice*, 2008. 39(4): pp. 381–388.

#21 Bonanno, G.A., "Loss, Trauma, and Human Resilience—Have We Underestimated the Human Capacity to Thrive After Extremely Aversive Events?" *American Psychologist*, 2004. 59(1): pp. 20–28.

#30 Burnell, K.J., P.G. Coleman, and N. Hunt, "Falklands War Veterans' Perceptions of Social Support and the Reconciliation of Traumatic Memories," *Aging & Mental Health*, 2006. 10(3): pp. 282–289.

#45 Eid, J., and B.H. Johnsen, "Acute Stress Reactions After Submarine Accidents," *Military Medicine*, 2002. 167(5): pp. 427–431.

#62 Hoge, E.A., E.D. Austin, and M.H. Pollack, "Resilience: Research Evidence and Conceptual Considerations for Posttraumatic Stress Disorder," *Depression and Anxiety*, 2007. 24(2): pp. 139–152.

#98 Peres, J.F.P., et al., "Spirituality and Resilience in Trauma Victims," *Journal of Religion & Health*, 2007. 46(3): pp. 343–350.

#118 Tiet, Q.Q., et al., "Coping, Symptoms, and Functioning Outcomes of Patients with Posttraumatic Stress Disorder," *Journal of Traumatic Stress*, 2006. 19(6): pp. 799–811.

#149 Wald, J., et al., *Literature Review of Concepts: Psychological Resiliency*. 2006, British Columbia University: Vancouver, Canada. p. 134.

#152 Black, K., and M. Lobo, "A Conceptual Review of Family Resilience Factors," *Journal of Family Nursing*, 2008. 14(1): pp. 33–55.

#155 Earvolino-Ramirez, M., "Resilience: A Concept Analysis," *Nursing Forum*, 2007. 42(2): pp. 73–82.

#164 Walsh, F., "Family Resilience: A Framework for Clinical Practice," *Family Process*, 2003. 42(1).

#166 Ritchie, B.S., P.J. Watson, and M.J. Friedman, eds. *Interventions Following Mass Violence and Disasters: Strategies for Mental Health Practice,* 2006, Guilford Press: New York.

#169 Nucifora, F., et al., *Building Resistance, Resilience, and Recovery in the Wake of School and Workplace Violence*. 2007, Department of Psychiatry and Behavioral Health Sciences, Johns Hopkins University School of Medicine.

#172 King, D.W., D.S. Vogt, and L.A. King, "Risk and Resilience Factors in the Etiology of Chronic Posttraumatic Stress Disorder," in *Early Intervention for Trauma and Traumatic Loss*, B. Litz, Editor. 2004, Guilford Press: New York, NY.

#178 Conger, R.D., and K.J. Conger, "Resilience in Midwestern Families: Selected Findings from the First Decade of a Prospective, Longitudinal Study," *Journal of Marriage and Family*, 2002. 64(2): pp. 361–373.

#191 Beardslee, W.R., "Resilience in Action," in *Out of the Darkened Room: When a Parent Is Depressed: Protecting the Children and Strengthening the Family*, 2002, Little, Brown: Boston.

#195 Aisenberg, E., and T. Herrenkohl, "Community Violence in Context: Risk and Resilience in Children and Families," *Journal of Interpersonal Violence*, 2008. 23(3): pp. 296–315.

#201 Ano, G.G., and E.B. Vasconcelles, "Religious Coping and Psychological Adjustment to Stress: A Meta-Analysis," *Journal of Clinical Psychology*, 2005. 61(4): pp. 461–480.

#216 Fredrickson, B.L., "The Role of Positive Emotions in Positive Psychology: The Broaden-and-Build Theory of Positive Emotions," *American Psychologist*, 2001. 56(3): pp. 218–226.

#230 Wiens, T.W., and P. Boss, "Maintaining Family Resiliency Before, During, and After Military Separation," in *Military Life: The Psychology of Serving in Peace and Combat*, T.W. Britt, A.B. Adler, and C.A. Castro, Editors. 2006, Praeger Security International: Westport, Conn.

#245 Hobfoll, S.E., et al., "Five Essential Elements of Immediate and Mid-Term Mass Trauma Intervention: Empirical Evidence," *Psychiatry*, 2007. 70(4): pp. 283–315.

#246 Masten, A.S., "Ordinary Magic: Resilience Processes in Development," *American Psychologist*, 2001. 56(3): pp. 227–238.

#248 Conger, R.D., M.A. Rueter, and G.H.J. Elder, "Couple Resilience to Economic Pressure," *Journal of Personality and Social Psychology*, 1999. 76(1): pp. 54–71.

#254 Haglund, M.E.M., et al., "Psychobiological Mechanisms of Resilience: Relevance to Prevention and Treatment of Stress-Related Psychopathology," *Development and Psychopathology*, 2007. 19: pp. 889–920.

#271 Campbell, D., K. Campbell, and J. Ness, "Resilience Through Leadership," in *Biobehavioral Resilience to Stress*, B.J. Lukey and V. Tepe, Editors. 2008, CRC Press: Boca Raton, Fla.

#274 Staal, M., et al., "Cognitive Performance and Resilience to Stress," in *Biobehavioral Resilience to Stress*, B.J. Lukey and V. Tepe, Editors. 2008, CRC Press: Boca Raton, Fla.

#277 Tugade, M.M., and B.L. Fredrickson, "Resilient Individuals Use Positive Emotions to Bounce Back from Negative Emotional Experiences," *Journal of Personality and Social Psychology*, 2004. 86(2): pp. 320–333.

#292 Solomon, Z., M. Mikulincer, and E. Avitzur, "Coping, Locus of Control, Social Support, and Combat-Related Posttraumatic Stress Disorder: A Prospective Study," *Journal of Personality and Social Psychology*, 1988. 55(2): pp. 279–285.

#294 Fredrickson, B.L., "Cultivating Positive Emotions to Optimize Health and Well-Being," *Prevention and Treatment*, 2000. 3(1).

#295 Butler, L.D., L.A. Morland, and G.A. Leskin, "Psychological Resilience in the Face of Terrorism," in *Psychology of Terrorism*, Bonger, et al., Editors. 2007, Oxford University Press: Oxford UK.

#314 Yehuda, R., et al., "Developing an Agenda for Translational Studies of Resilience and Vulnerability Following Trauma Exposure," *New York Academy of Sciences*, 2006. 1071: pp. 379–396.

#321 Gillham, J.E., et al., "School-Based Prevention of Depressive Symptoms: A Randomized Controlled Study of the Effectiveness and Specificity of the Penn Resilience Program," *Journal of Consulting and Clinical Psychology*, 2007. 75(1): pp. 9–19.

#325 Maddi, S.R., "Relevance of Hardiness Assessment and Training to the Military Context," *Military Psychology*, 2007. 19(1): pp. 61–70.

#329 Zach, S., S. Raviv, and R. Inbar, "The Benefits of a Graduated Training Program for Security Officers on Physical Performance in Stressful Situations," *International Journal of Stress Management*, 2007. 14(4): pp. 350–369.

#330 Williams, A., et al., "Psychosocial Effects of the Boot Strap Intervention in Navy Recruits," *Military Medicine*, 2004. 169(10): pp. 814–820.

#332 Gill, Jessica, et al., *Dispositional Traits and Social Factors Related to Trauma Resilience: Implications for Therapy*, unpublished manuscript, 2010.

#343 Tiller, W.A., R. McCraty, and M. Atkinson, "Cardiac Coherence: A New, Noninvasive Measure of Autonomic Nervous System Order," *Alternative Therapies*, 1996. 2(1): pp. 52–65.

#353 Stanley, E.A., et al., "Mind Fitness in Counterinsurgency: Addressing the Cognitive Requirements of Population-Centric Operations," *Military Review*, 2010. 90(1).

#354 Stanley, E.A., "Neuroplasticity, Mind Fitness, and Military Effectiveness," in *The "New" Biological Warfare: Biotechnology and the Future of America's Military*, M. Drapeau, Editor. 2009, National Defense University Press: Washington, D.C.

Positive Affect

#2 Gelkopf, M., et al., "The Impact of 'Training the Trainers' Course for Helping Tsunami-Survivor Children on Sri Lankan Disaster Volunteer Workers," *International Journal of Stress Management*, 2008. 15(2): pp. 117–135.

#3 Vernberg, E.M., et al., "Innovations in Disaster Mental Health: Psychological First Aid," *Professional Psychology: Research and Practice*, 2008. 39(4): pp. 381–388.

#6 Van Vliet, K.J., "Shame and Resilience in Adulthood: A Grounded Theory Study," *Journal of Counseling Psychology*, 2008. 55(2): pp. 233–245.

#21 Bonanno, G.A., "Loss, Trauma, and Human Resilience—Have We Underestimated the Human Capacity to Thrive After Extremely Aversive Events?" *American Psychologist*, 2004. 59(1): pp. 20–28.

#62 Hoge, E.A., E.D. Austin, and M.H. Pollack, "Resilience: Research Evidence and Conceptual Considerations for Posttraumatic Stress Disorder," *Depression and Anxiety*, 2007. 24(2): pp. 139–152.

#65 Jennings, P.A., et al., "Combat Exposure, Perceived Benefits of Military Service, and Wisdom in Later Life—Findings from the Normative Aging Study," *Research on Aging*, 2006. 28(1): pp. 115–134.

#81 Maguen, S., et al., "Description of Risk and Resilience Factors Among Military Medical Personnel Before Deployment to Iraq," *Military Medicine*, 2008. 173(1): pp. 1–9.

#144 Thompson, M.M. and M.A. Gignac, *A Model of Psychological Adaptation in Peace Support Operations: An Overview*. 2001, Defence and Civil Institute of Environmental Medicine: Downsview, Ontario—Canada. p. 50.

#149 Wald, J., et al., *Literature Review of Concepts: Psychological Resiliency*. 2006, British Columbia University: Vancouver, Canada. p. 134.

#152 Black, K., and M. Lobo, "A Conceptual Review of Family Resilience Factors," *Journal of Family Nursing*, 2008. 14(1): pp. 33–55.

#155 Earvolino-Ramirez, M., "Resilience: A Concept Analysis," *Nursing Forum*, 2007. 42(2): pp. 73–82.

#156 Fredrickson, B.L., et al., "What Good Are Positive Emotions in Crises? A Prospective Study of Resilience and Emotions Following the Terrorist Attacks on the United States on September 11th, 2001," *Journal of Personality and Social Psychology*, 2003. 84(2): pp. 365–376.

#164 Walsh, F., "Family Resilience: A Framework for Clinical Practice," *Family Process*, 2003. 42(1).

#166 Ritchie, B.S., P.J. Watson, and M.J. Friedman, eds. *Interventions Following Mass Violence and Disasters: Strategies for Mental Health Practice*. 2006, Guilford Press: New York.

#216 Fredrickson, B.L., "The Role of Positive Emotions in Positive Psychology: The Broaden-and-Build Theory of Positive Emotions," *American Psychologist*, 2001. 56(3): pp. 218–226.

#226 Hoge, C.W., et al., "Combat Duty in Iraq and Afghanistan, Mental Health Problems, and Barriers to Care," *New England Journal of Medicine*, 2004. 351(1): pp. 13–22.

#229 Tusaie, K., and J. Dyer, "Resilience: A Historical Review of the Construct," *Holist Nurs Pract*, 2004. 18(1): pp. 3–8.

#245 Hobfoll, S.E., et al., "Five Essential Elements of Immediate and Mid-Term Mass Trauma Intervention: Empirical Evidence," *Psychiatry*, 2007. 70(4): pp. 283–315.

#254 Haglund, M.E.M., et al., "Psychobiological Mechanisms of Resilience: Relevance to Prevention and Treatment of Stress-Related Psychopathology," *Development and Psychopathology*, 2007. 19: pp. 889–920.

#263 Hjemdal, O., et al., "Predicting Psychiatric Symptoms," *Clinical Psychology and Psychotherapy*, 2006. 13: pp. 194–201.

#272 Southwick, S., et al., "Adaptation to Stress and Psychobiological Mechanisms of Resilience," in *Biobehavioral Resilience to Stress*, B.J. Lukey and V. Tepe, Editors. 2008, CRC Press: Boca Raton, FL.

#277 Tugade, M.M., and B.L. Fredrickson, "Resilient Individuals Use Positive Emotions to Bounce Back from Negative Emotional Experiences," *Journal of Personality and Social Psychology*, 2004. 86(2): pp. 320–333.

#294 Fredrickson, B.L., "Cultivating Positive Emotions to Optimize Health and Well-Being," *Prevention and Treatment*, 2000. 3(1).

#295 Butler, L.D., L.A. Morland, and G.A. Leskin, "Psychological Resilience in the Face of Terrorism," in *Psychology of Terrorism*, Bonger, et al., Editors. 2007, Oxford University Press: Oxford, UK.

#312 Smith, L.M., and J.M. Violanti, "Risk Response Model," in *Promoting Capabilities to Manage Posttraumatic Stress*, D. Paton, J.M. Violanti, and L.M. Smith, Editors. 2003, Charles C. Thomas Publisher, Ltd.: Springfield, Illinois.

#314 Yehuda, R., et al., "Developing an Agenda for Translational Studies of Resilience and Vulnerability Following Trauma Exposure," *New York Academy of Sciences*, 2006. 1071: pp. 379–396.

#321 Gillham, J.E., et al., "School-Based Prevention of Depressive Symptoms: A Randomized Controlled Study of the Effectiveness and Specificity of the Penn Resilience Program," *Journal of Consulting and Clinical Psychology*, 2007. 75(1): pp. 9–19.

#332 Gill, Jessica, et al., *Dispositional Traits and Social Factors Related to Trauma Resilience: Implications for Therapy*, unpublished manuscript, 2010.

#343 Tiller, W.A., R. McCraty, and M. Atkinson, "Cardiac Coherence: A New, Noninvasive Measure of Autonomic Nervous System Order," *Alternative Therapies*, 1996. 2(1): pp. 52–65.

#344 Luskin, F., et al., "A Controlled Pilot Study of Stress Management Training of Elderly Patients with Congestive Heart Failure," *Preventive Cardiology*, 2002(Fall): pp. 168–176.

#345 McCraty, R., et al., "The Effects of Emotions on Short-Term Power Spectrum Analysis of Heart Rate Variability," *American Journal of Cardiology*, 1995. 76(4): pp. 1089–1093.

#346 McCraty, R., M. Atkinson, and D. Tomasino, "Impact of Workplace Stress Reduction Program on Blood Pressure and Emotional Health in Hypertensive Employees," *Journal of Alternative and Complementary Medicine*, 2003. 9(3): pp. 355–369.

#347 Rozman, D., et al., "A Pilot Intervention Program That Reduced Psychological Symptomatology in Individuals with Human Immunodeficiency Virus," *Complementary Therapies in Medicine*, 1996. 4: pp. 226–232.

#350 McCraty, R., et al., "The Impact of a New Emotional Self-Management Program on Stress, Emotions, Heart Rate Variability, DHEA and Cortisol," *Integrative Physiological and Behavioral Science*, 1998. 33(2): pp. 151–170.

#351 McCraty, R., et al., "Hew Hope for Correctional Officers: An Innovative Program for Reducing Stress and Health Risks," *Applied Psychophysiology and Biofeedback*, 2009. 34(4).

#353 Stanley, E.A., et al., "Mind Fitness in Counterinsurgency: Addressing the Cognitive Requirements of Population-Centric Operations." *Military Review*, 2010. 90(1).

Positive Thinking

#2 Gelkopf, M., et al., "The Impact of 'Training the Trainers' Course for Helping Tsunami-Survivor Children on Sri Lankan Disaster Volunteer Workers," *International Journal of Stress Management*, 2008. 15(2): pp. 117–135.

#3 Vernberg, E.M., et al., "Innovations in Disaster Mental Health: Psychological First Aid," *Professional Psychology: Research and Practice*, 2008. 39(4): pp. 381–388.

#51 Friedman, M., and C. Higson-Smith, "Building Psychological Resilience: Learning from the South African Police Service," in *Promoting Capabilities to Manage Posttraumatic Stress: Perspectives on Resilience*, D. Paton, J.M. Violanti, and L.M. Smith, Editors. 2003, Charles C. Thomas: Springfield, Illinois. pp. 103–118.

#62 Hoge, E.A., E.D. Austin, and M.H. Pollack, "Resilience: Research Evidence and Conceptual Considerations for Posttraumatic Stress Disorder," *Depression and Anxiety*, 2007. 24(2): pp. 139–152.

#65 Jennings, P.A., et al., "Combat Exposure, Perceived Benefits of Military Service, and Wisdom in Later Life—Findings from the Normative Aging Study," *Research on Aging*, 2006. 28(1): pp. 115–134.

#144 Thompson, M.M., and M.A. Gignac, *A Model of Psychological Adaptation in Peace Support Operations: An Overview*. 2001, Defence and Civil Institute of Environmental Medicine: Downsview, Ontario—Canada. p. 50.

#145 Thompson, M.M., and D.R. McCreary, *Enhancing Mental Readiness in Military Personnel*. 2006, Defence Research and Development: Toronto, Canada. p. 13.

#149 Wald, J., et al., *Literature Review of Concepts: Psychological Resiliency*. 2006, British Columbia University: Vancouver, Canada. p. 134.

#152 Black, K., and M. Lobo, "A Conceptual Review of Family Resilience Factors," *Journal of Family Nursing*, 2008. 14(1): pp. 33–55.

#156 Fredrickson, B.L., et al., "What Good Are Positive Emotions in Crises? A Prospective Study of Resilience and Emotions Following the Terrorist Attacks on the United States on September 11th, 2001," *Journal of Personality and Social Psychology*, 2003. 84(2): pp. 365–376.

#159 MacDermid, S.M., et al., *Understanding and Promoting Resilience in Military Families*. 2008, Military Family Research Institute at Purdue Univeristy: West Lafayette.

#164 Walsh, F., "Family Resilience: A Framework for Clinical Practice," *Family Process*, 2003. 42(1).

#166 Ritchie, B.S., P.J. Watson, and M.J. Friedman, eds. *Interventions Following Mass Violence and Disasters: Strategies for Mental Health Practice*. 2006, Guilford Press: New York.

#169 Nucifora, F., et al., *Building Resistance, Resilience, and Recovery in the Wake of School and Workplace Violence*. 2007, Department of Psychiatry and Behavioral Health Sciences, Johns Hopkins University School of Medicine.

#174 Bartone, P.T., "Resilience Under Military Operational Stress: Can Leaders Influence Hardiness?" *Military Psychology*, 2006. 18(3 supp 1): pp. 131–148.

#188 Coleman, M., and L. Ganong, "Resilience and Families," *Family Relations*, 2002. 51(2): pp. 101–102.

#201 Ano, G.G., and E.B. Vasconcelles, "Religious Coping and Psychological Adjustment to Stress: A Meta-Analysis," *Journal of Clinical Psychology*, 2005. 61(4): pp. 461–480.

#218 Paton, D., "Critical Incident Stress Risk in Police Officers: Managing Resilience and Vulnerability," *Traumatology*, 2006. 12(198): pp. 198–205.

#226 Hoge, C.W., et al., "Combat Duty in Iraq and Afghanistan, Mental Health Problems, and Barriers to Care," *New England Journal of Medicine*, 2004. 351(1): pp. 13–22.

#229 Tusaie, K., and J. Dyer, "Resilience: A Historical Review of the Construct," *Holist Nurs Pract*, 2004. 18(1): pp. 3–8.

#245 Hobfoll, S.E., et al., "Five Essential Elements of Immediate and Mid-Term Mass Trauma Intervention: Empirical Evidence," *Psychiatry*, 2007. 70(4): pp. 283–315.

#246 Masten, A.S., "Ordinary Magic: Resilience Processes in Development," *American Psychologist*, 2001. 56(3): pp. 227–238.

#254 Haglund, M.E.M., et al., "Psychobiological Mechanisms of Resilience: Relevance to Prevention and Treatment of Stress-Related Psychopathology," *Development and Psychopathology*, 2007. 19: pp. 889–920.

#263 Hjemdal, O., et al., "Predicting Psychiatric Symptoms," *Clinical Psychology and Psychotherapy*, 2006. 13: pp. 194–201.

#271 Campbell, D., K. Campbell, and J. Ness, "Resilience Through Leadership," in *Biobehavioral Resilience to Stress*, B.J. Lukey and V. Tepe, Editors. 2008, CRC Press: Boca Raton, FL.

#277 Tugade, M.M., and B.L. Fredrickson, "Resilient Individuals Use Positive Emotions to Bounce Back from Negative Emotional Experiences," *Journal of Personality and Social Psychology*, 2004. 86(2): pp. 320–333.

#288 Taylor, S., "Adjustment to Threatening Events: A Theory of Cognitive Adaptation," *American Psychologist*, 1983(November): pp. 1161–1173.

#293 Affleck, G., and H. Tennen, "Construing Benefits from Adversity: Adaptational Significance and Dispositional Underpinnings," *Journal of Personality*, 1996. 64(4): pp. 899–922.

294 Fredrickson, B.L., "Cultivating Positive Emotions to Optimize Health and Well-Being," *Prevention and Treatment*, 2000. 3(1).

295 Butler, L.D., L.A. Morland, and G.A. Leskin, "Psychological Resilience in the Face of Terrorism," in *Psychology of Terrorism*, Bonger, et al., Editors. 2007, Oxford University Press: Oxford, UK.

305 Bartone, P.T., "Hardiness as a Resiliency Resource Under High Stress Conditions," in *Promoting Capabilities to Manage Posttraumatic Stress*, D. Paton, J.M. Violanti, and L.M. Smith, Editors. 2003, Charles C. Thomas Publisher, Ltd.: Springfield, Illinois.

314 Yehuda, R., et al., "Developing an Agenda for Translational Studies of Resilience and Vulnerability Following Trauma Exposure," *New York Academy of Sciences*, 2006. 1071: pp. 379–396.

315 Calhoun, L.G., and R.G. Tedeschi, "Routes to Posttraumatic Growth Through Cognitive Processing," in *Promoting Capabilities to Manage Posttraumatic Stress*, D. Paton, J.M. Violanti, and L.M. Smith, Editors. 2003, Charles C. Thomas Publisher, Ltd.: Springfield, Illinois.

321 Gillham, J.E., et al., "School-Based Prevention of Depressive Symptoms: A Randomized Controlled Study of the Effectiveness and Specificity of the Penn Resilience Program," *Journal of Consulting and Clinical Psychology*, 2007. 75(1): pp. 9–19.

326 Morgan, C.A., et al., "Relation Between Cardiac Vagal Tone and Performance in Male Military Personnel Exposed to High Stress: Three Prospective Studies," *Psychophysiology*, 2007. 44: pp. 120–127.

332 Gill, Jessica, et al., *Dispositional Traits and Social Factors Related to Trauma Resilience: Implications for Therapy*, unpublished manuscript, 2010.

340 Adler, A.B., et al., "Battlemind Debriefing and Battlemind Training as Early Interventions with Soldiers Returning from Iraq: Randomized by Platoon," *Journal of Consulting and Clinical Psychology*, 2009. 77(5): pp. 928–940.

344 Luskin, F., et al., "A Controlled Pilot Study of Stress Management Training of Elderly Patients with Congestive Heart Failure," *Preventive Cardiology*, 2002(Fall): pp. 168–176.

346 McCraty, R., M. Atkinson, and D. Tomasino, "Impact of Workplace Stress Reduction Program on Blood Pressure and Emotional Health in Hypertensive Employees," *Journal of Alternative and Complementary Medicine*, 2003. 9(3): pp. 355–369.

350 McCraty, R., et al., "The Impact of a New Emotional Self-Management Program on Stress, Emotions, Heart Rate Variability, DHEA and Cortisol," *Integrative Physiological and Behavioral Science*, 1998. 33(2): pp. 151–170.

351 McCraty, R., et al., "New Hope for Correctional Officers: An Innovative Program for Reducing Stress and Health Risks," *Applied Psychophysiology and Biofeedback*, 2009. 34(4).

353 Stanley, E.A., et al., "Mind Fitness in Counterinsurgency: Addressing the Cognitive Requirements of Population-Centric Operations," *Military Review*, 2010. 90(1).

Realism

#2 Gelkopf, M., et al., "The Impact of 'Training the Trainers' Course for Helping Tsunami-Survivor Children on Sri Lankan Disaster Volunteer Workers," *International Journal of Stress Management*, 2008. 15(2): pp. 117–135.

#3 Vernberg, E.M., et al., "Innovations in Disaster Mental Health: Psychological First Aid," *Professional Psychology: Research and Practice*, 2008. 39(4): pp. 381–388.

#21 Bonanno, G.A., "Loss, Trauma, and Human Resilience—Have We Underestimated the Human Capacity to Thrive After Extremely Aversive Events?" *American Psychologist*, 2004. 59(1): pp. 20–28.

#62 Hoge, E.A., E.D. Austin, and M.H. Pollack, "Resilience: Research Evidence and Conceptual Considerations for Posttraumatic Stress Disorder," *Depression and Anxiety*, 2007. 24(2): pp. 139–152.

#144 Thompson, M.M., and M.A. Gignac, *A Model of Psychological Adaptation in Peace Support Operations: An Overview*. 2001, Defense and Civil Institute of Environmental Medicine: Downsview, Ontario—Canada. p. 50.

#149 Wald, J., et al., *Literature Review of Concepts: Psychological Resiliency*. 2006, British Columbia University: Vancouver, Canada. p. 134.

#155 Earvolino-Ramirez, M., "Resilience: A Concept Analysis," *Nursing Forum*, 2007. 42(2): pp. 73–82.

#159 MacDermid, S.M., et al., *Understanding and Promoting Resilience in Military Families*. 2008, Military Family Research Institute at Purdue University: West Lafayette.

#166 Ritchie, B.S., P.J. Watson, and M.J. Friedman, eds. *Interventions Following Mass Violence and Disasters: Strategies for Mental Health Practice*. 2006, Guilford Press: New York.

#169 Nucifora, F., et al., *Building Resistance, Resilience, and Recovery in the Wake of School and Workplace Violence*. 2007, Department of Psychiatry and Behavioral Health Sciences, Johns Hopkins University School of Medicine.

#178 Conger, R.D., and K.J. Conger, "Resilience in Midwestern Families: Selected Findings from the First Decade of a Prospective, Longitudinal Study," *Journal of Marriage and Family*, 2002. 64(2): pp. 361–373.

#201 Ano, G.G., and E.B. Vasconcelles, "Religious Coping and Psychological Adjustment to Stress: A Meta-Analysis," *Journal of Clinical Psychology*, 2005. 61(4): pp. 461–480.

#206 Fraley, R.C., et al., "Attachment and Psychological Adaptation in High Exposure Survivors of the September 11th Attack on the World Trade Center," *Personality and Social Psychology Bulletin*, 2006. 32.

#223 Barton, W., "Methodological Challenges in the Study of Resilience," in *Handbook for Working with Children and Youth: Pathways to Resilience Across Cultures and Contexts*, M. Ungar, Editor. 2003, Sage Publications: Thousand Oaks, CA. pp. 135–147.

#226 Hoge, C.W., et al., "Combat Duty in Iraq and Afghanistan, Mental Health Problems, and Barriers to Care," *New England Journal of Medicine*, 2004. 351(1): pp. 13–22.

#228 Luthar, S.S., and D. Cicchetti, "The Construct of Resilience: Implications for Interventions and Social Policies," *Developmental Psychopathology*, 2000. 12(4): pp. 857–885.

#229 Tusaie, K., and J. Dyer, "Resilience: A Historical Review of the Construct," *Holist Nurs Pract*, 2004. 18(1): pp. 3–8.

#245 Hobfoll, S.E., et al., "Five Essential Elements of Immediate and Mid-Term Mass Trauma Intervention: Empirical Evidence," *Psychiatry*, 2007. 70(4): pp. 283–315.

#288 Taylor, S., "Adjustment to Threatening Events: A Theory of Cognitive Adaptation," *American Psychologist*, 1983(November): pp. 1161–1173.

#292 Solomon, Z., M. Mikulincer, and E. Avitzur, "Coping, Locus of Control, Social Support, and Combat-Related Posttraumatic Stress Disorder: A Prospective Study," *Journal of Personality and Social Psychology*, 1988. 55(2): pp. 279–285.

294 Fredrickson, B.L., "Cultivating Positive Emotions to Optimize Health and Well-Being," *Prevention and Treatment*, 2000. 3(1).

295 Butler, L.D., L.A. Morland, and G.A. Leskin, "Psychological Resilience in the Face of Terrorism," in *Psychology of Terrorism*, Bonger, et al., Editors. 2007, Oxford University Press: Oxford, UK.

314 Yehuda, R., et al., "Developing an Agenda for Translational Studies of Resilience and Vulnerability Following Trauma Exposure," *New York Academy of Sciences*, 2006. 1071: pp. 379–396.

321 Gillham, J.E., et al., "School-Based Prevention of Depressive Symptoms: A Randomized Controlled Study of the Effectiveness and Specificity of the Penn Resilience Program," *Journal of Consulting and Clinical Psychology*, 2007. 75(1): pp. 9–19.

325 Maddi, S.R., "Relevance of Hardiness Assessment and Training to the Military Context," *Military Psychology*, 2007. 19(1): pp. 61–70.

329 Zach, S., S. Raviv, and R. Inbar, "The Benefits of a Graduated Training Program for Security Officers on Physical Performance in Stressful Situations," *International Journal of Stress Management*, 2007. 14(4): pp. 350–369.

332 Gill, Jessica, et al., *Dispositional Traits and Social Factors Related to Trauma Resilience: Implications for Therapy*, unpublished manuscript, 2010.

343 Tiller, W.A., R. McCraty, and M. Atkinson, "Cardiac Coherence: A New, Noninvasive Measure of Autonomic Nervous System Order," *Alternative Therapies*, 1996. 2(1): pp. 52–65.

353 Stanley, E.A., et al., "Mind Fitness in Counterinsurgency: Addressing the Cognitive Requirements of Population-Centric Operations," *Military Review*, 2010. 90(1).

Behavioral Control

#3 Vernberg, E.M., et al., "Innovations in Disaster Mental Health: Psychological First Aid," *Professional Psychology: Research and Practice*, 2008. 39(4): pp. 381–388.

#23 Bonanno, G.A., et al., "What Predicts Psychological Resilience After Disaster? The Role of Demographics, Resources, and Life Stress," *Journal of Consulting and Clinical Psychology*, 2007. 75(5): pp. 671–682.

#24 Bonanno, G.A., C. Rennicke, and S. Dekel, "Self-Enhancement Among High-Exposure Survivors of the September 11th Terrorist Attack: Resilience or Social Maladjustment?" *Journal of Personality and Social Psychology*, 2005. 88(6): pp. 984–998.

#149 Wald, J., et al., *Literature Review of Concepts: Psychological Resiliency*. 2006, British Columbia University: Vancouver, Canada. p. 134.

#155 Earvolino-Ramirez, M., "Resilience: A Concept Analysis," *Nursing Forum*, 2007. 42(2): pp. 73–82.

#159 MacDermid, S.M., et al., *Understanding and Promoting Resilience in Military Families*. 2008, Military Family Research Institute at Purdue University: West Lafayette.

#189 Hipke, K.N., et al., "Predictors of Children's Intervention-Induced Resilience in a Parenting Program for Divorced Mothers," *Family Relations*, 2002. 51(2): pp. 121–129.

#209 Scarpa, A., S.C. Haden, and J. Hurley, "Community Violence Victimization and Symptoms of Posttraumatic Stress Disorder: The Moderating Effects of Coping and Social Support," *Journal of Interpersonal Violence*, 2006. 21: pp. 446–469.

#243 O'Donnell, D.A., M.E. Schwab-Stone, and A.Z. Muyeed, "Multidimensional Resilience in Urban Children Exposed to Community Violence," *Child Development*, 2002. 73(4): pp. 1265–1282.

#246 Masten, A.S., "Ordinary Magic: Resilience Processes in Development," *American Psychologist*, 2001. 56(3): pp. 227–238.

#314 Yehuda, R., et al., "Developing an Agenda for Translational Studies of Resilience and Vulnerability Following Trauma Exposure," *New York Academy of Sciences*, 2006. 1071: pp. 379–396.

#321 Gillham, J.E., et al., "School-Based Prevention of Depressive Symptoms: A Randomized Controlled Study of the Effectiveness and Specificity of the Penn Resilience Program," *Journal of Consulting and Clinical Psychology*, 2007. 75(1): pp. 9–19.

#326 Morgan, C.A., et al., "Relation Between Cardiac Vagal Tone and Performance in Male Military Personnel Exposed to High Stress: Three Prospective Studies," *Psychophysiology*, 2007. 44: pp. 120–127.

#347 Rozman, D., et al., "A Pilot Intervention Program That Reduced Psychological Symptomatology in Individuals with Human Immunodeficiency Virus," *Complementary Therapies in Medicine*, 1996. 4: pp. 226–232.

#348 McCraty, R., et al., "The Impact of an Emotional Self-Management Skills Course on Psychosocial Functioning and Autonomic Recovery to Stress in Middle School Children," *Integrative Physiological and Behavioral Science*, 1999. 34(4): pp. 246–268.

#351 McCraty, R., et al., "Hew Hope for Correctional Officers: An Innovative Program for Reducing Stress and Health Risks," *Applied Psychophysiology and Biofeedback*, 2009. 34(4).

#353 Stanley, E.A., et al., "Mind Fitness in Counterinsurgency: Addressing the Cognitive Requirements of Population-Centric Operations," *Military Review*, 2010. 90(1).

#354 Stanley, E.A., "Neuroplasticity, Mind Fitness, and Military Effectiveness," in *The "New" Biological Warfare: Biotechnology and the Future of America's Military*, M. Drapeau, Editor. 2009, National Defense University Press: Washington, D.C.

Physical Fitness

#95 Palmer, C., "A Theory of Risk and Resilience Factors in Military Families," *Military Psychology*, 2008. 20(3): pp. 205–217.

#166 Ritchie, B.S., P.J. Watson, and M.J. Friedman, eds. *Interventions Following Mass Violence and Disasters: Strategies for Mental Health Practice*. 2006, Guilford Press: New York.

#325 Maddi, S.R., "Relevance of Hardiness Assessment and Training to the Military Context," *Military Psychology*, 2007. 19(1): pp. 61–70.

#351 McCraty, R., et al., "New Hope for Correctional Officers: An Innovative Program for Reducing Stress and Health Risks," *Applied Psychophysiology and Biofeedback*, 2009. 34(4).

Altruism

#254 Haglund, M.E.M., et al., "Psychobiological Mechanisms of Resilience: Relevance to Prevention and Treatment of Stress-Related Psychopathology," *Development and Psychopathology*, 2007. 19: pp. 889–920.

Family-Level Factors

Emotional Ties

#62 Hoge, E.A., E.D. Austin, and M.H. Pollack, "Resilience: Research Evidence and Conceptual Considerations for Posttraumatic Stress Disorder," *Depression and Anxiety*, 2007. 24(2): pp. 139–152.

#152 Black, K., and M. Lobo, "A Conceptual Review of Family Resilience Factors," *Journal of Family Nursing*, 2008. 14(1): pp. 33–55.

#178 Conger, R.D., and K.J. Conger, "Resilience in Midwestern Families: Selected Findings from the First Decade of a Prospective, Longitudinal Study," *Journal of Marriage and Family*, 2002. 64(2): pp. 361–373.

#195 Aisenberg, E., and T. Herrenkohl, "Community Violence in Context: Risk and Resilience in Children and Families," *Journal of Interpersonal Violence*, 2008. 23(3): pp. 296–315.

#250 Vogt, D.S., and L.R. Tanner, "Risk and Resilience Factors for Posttraumatic Stress Symptomatology in Gulf War I Veterans," *Journal of Traumatic Stress*, 2007. 20(1): pp. 27–38.

#318 Bell, C.C., "Cultivating Resiliency in Youth," *Journal of Adolescent Health*, 2001. 29: pp. 375–381.

Communication

#152 Black, K., and M. Lobo, "A Conceptual Review of Family Resilience Factors," *Journal of Family Nursing*, 2008. 14(1): pp. 33–55.

#159 MacDermid, S.M., et al., *Understanding and Promoting Resilience in Military Families*. 2008, Military Family Research Institute at Purdue University: West Lafayette.

#169 Nucifora, F., et al., *Building Resistance, Resilience, and Recovery in the Wake of School and Workplace Violence*. 2007, Department of Psychiatry and Behavioral Health Sciences, Johns Hopkins University School of Medicine.

#240 Van Breda, A.D., *Resilience Theory: A Literature Review*. 2001, South African Military Health Service, Military Psychological Institute, Social Work Research & Development: Pretoria, South Africa.

#243 O'Donnell, D.A., M.E. Schwab-Stone, and A.Z. Muyeed, "Multidimensional Resilience in Urban Children Exposed to Community Violence," *Child Development*, 2002. 73(4): pp. 1265–1282.

#278 Pfefferbaum, B., et al., "Building Resilience to Mass Trauma Events," in *Handbook on Injury and Violence Prevention*, L.S. Doll, et al., Editors. 2007, Centers for Disease Control and Prevention, National Center for Injury Prevention and Control: Atlanta, GA.

#318 Bell, C.C., "Cultivating Resiliency in Youth," *Journal of Adolescent Health*, 2001. 29: pp. 375–381.

#321 Gillham, J.E., et al., "School-Based Prevention of Depressive Symptoms: A Randomized Controlled Study of the Effectiveness and Specificity of the Penn Resilience Program," *Journal of Consulting and Clinical Psychology*, 2007. 75(1): pp. 9–19.

#351 McCraty, R., et al., "New Hope for Correctional Officers: An Innovative Program for Reducing Stress and Health Risks," *Applied Psychophysiology and Biofeedback*, 2009. 34(4).

Support

#152 Black, K., and M. Lobo, "A Conceptual Review of Family Resilience Factors," *Journal of Family Nursing*, 2008. 14(1): pp. 33–55.

#166 Ritchie, B.S., P.J. Watson, and M.J. Friedman, eds. *Interventions Following Mass Violence and Disasters: Strategies for Mental Health Practice*. 2006, Guilford Press: New York.

#178 Conger, R.D., and K.J. Conger, "Resilience in Midwestern Families: Selected Findings from the First Decade of a Prospective, Longitudinal Study," *Journal of Marriage and Family*, 2002. 64(2): pp. 361–373.

#187 Letourneau, N., et al., "Supporting Parents: Can Intervention Improve Parent-Child Relationships?" *Journal of Family Nursing*, 2001. 7(2): pp. 159–187.

#188 Coleman, M., and L. Ganong, "Resilience and Families," *Family Relations*, 2002. 51(2): pp. 101–102.

#195 Aisenberg, E., and T. Herrenkohl, "Community Violence in Context: Risk and Resilience in Children and Families," *Journal of Interpersonal Violence*, 2008. 23(3): pp. 296–315.

#197 Barbarin, O.A., L. Richter, and T. deWet, "Exposure to Violence, Coping Resources, and Psychological Adjustment of South African Children," *American Journal of Orthopsychiatry*, 2001. 71(1).

#209 Scarpa, A., S.C. Haden, and J. Hurley, "Community Violence Victimization and Symptoms of Posttraumatic Stress Disorder: The Moderating Effects of Coping and Social Support," *Journal of Interpersonal Violence*, 2006. 21: pp. 446–469.

#212 Condly, S.J., "Resilience in Children: A Review of Literature with Implications for Education," *Urban Education*, 2006. 41: pp. 211–236.

#218 Paton, D., "Critical Incident Stress Risk in Police Officers: Managing Resilience and Vulnerability," *Traumatology*, 2006. 12(198): pp. 198–205.

#223 Barton, W., "Methodological Challenges in the Study of Resilience," in *Handbook for Working with Children and Youth: Pathways to Resilience Across Cultures and Contexts*, M. Ungar, Editor. 2003, Sage Publications: Thousand Oaks, CA. pp. 135–147.

#240 Van Breda, A.D., *Resilience Theory: A Literature Review*. 2001, South African Military Health Service, Military Psychological Institute, Social Work Research & Development: Pretoria, South Africa.

#243 O'Donnell, D.A., M.E. Schwab-Stone, and A.Z. Muyeed, "Multidimensional Resilience in Urban Children Exposed to Community Violence," *Child Development*, 2002. 73(4): pp. 1265–1282.

#248 Conger, R.D., M.A. Rueter, and G.H.J. Elder, "Couple Resilience to Economic Pressure," *Journal of Personality and Social Psychology*, 1999. 76(1): pp. 54–71.

#278 Pfefferbaum, B., et al., "Building Resilience to Mass Trauma Events," in *Handbook on Injury and Violence Prevention*, L.S. Doll, et al., Editors. 2007, Centers for Disease Control and Prevention, National Center for Injury Prevention and Control: Atlanta, GA.

#314 Yehuda, R., et al., "Developing an Agenda for Translational Studies of Resilience and Vulnerability Following Trauma Exposure," *New York Academy of Sciences*, 2006. 1071: pp. 379–396.

#318 Bell, C.C., "Cultivating Resiliency in Youth," *Journal of Adolescent Health*, 2001. 29: pp. 375–381.

#325 Maddi, S.R., "Relevance of Hardiness Assessment and Training to the Military Context," *Military Psychology*, 2007. 19(1): pp. 61–70.

332 Gill, Jessica, et al., *Dispositional Traits and Social Factors Related to Trauma Resilience: Implications for Therapy*, unpublished manuscript, 2010.

Closeness

159 MacDermid, S.M., et al., *Understanding and Promoting Resilience in Military Families*. 2008, Military Family Research Institute at Purdue University: West Lafayette.

314 Yehuda, R., et al., "Developing an Agenda for Translational Studies of Resilience and Vulnerability Following Trauma Exposure," *New York Academy of Sciences*, 2006. 1071: pp. 379–396.

318 Bell, C.C., "Cultivating Resiliency in Youth," *Journal of Adolescent Health*, 2001. 29: pp. 375–381.

330 Williams, A., et al., "Psychosocial Effects of the Boot Strap Intervention in Navy Recruits," *Military Medicine*, 2004. 169(10): pp. 814–820.

Nurturing

101 Qouta, S., et al., "Predictors of Psychological Distress and Positive Resources Among Palestinian Adolescents: Trauma, Child, and Mothering Characteristics," *Child Abuse and Neglect*, 2007. 31(7): pp. 699–717.

*159 MacDermid, S.M., et al., *Understanding and Promoting Resilience in Military Families*. 2008, Military Family Research Institute at Purdue University: West Lafayette.

*166 Ritchie, B.S., P.J. Watson, and M.J. Friedman, eds. *Interventions Following Mass Violence and Disasters: Strategies for Mental Health Practice*. 2006, Guilford Press: New York.

*178 Conger, R.D., and K.J. Conger, "Resilience in Midwestern Families: Selected Findings from the First Decade of a Prospective, Longitudinal Study," *Journal of Marriage and Family*, 2002. 64(2): pp. 361–373.

*187 Letourneau, N., et al., "Supporting Parents: Can Intervention Improve Parent-Child Relationships?" *Journal of Family Nursing*, 2001. 7(2): pp. 159–187.

*188 Coleman, M., and L. Ganong, "Resilience and Families," *Family Relations*, 2002. 51(2): pp. 101–102.

*223 Barton, W., "Methodological Challenges in the Study of Resilience," in *Handbook for Working with Children and Youth: Pathways to Resilience Across Cultures and Contexts*, M. Ungar, Editor. 2003, Sage Publications: Thousand Oaks, CA. pp. 135–147.

*243 O'Donnell, D.A., M.E. Schwab-Stone, and A.Z. Muyeed, "Multidimensional Resilience in Urban Children Exposed to Community Violence," *Child Development*, 2002. 73(4): pp. 1265–1282.

*246 Masten, A.S., "Ordinary Magic: Resilience Processes in Development," *American Psychologist*, 2001. 56(3): pp. 227–238.

*318 Bell, C.C., "Cultivating Resiliency in Youth," *Journal of Adolescent Health*, 2001. 29: pp. 375–381.

Adaptability

*152 Black, K., and M. Lobo, "A Conceptual Review of Family Resilience Factors," *Journal of Family Nursing*, 2008. 14(1): pp. 33–55.

*196 Patterson, J.M., "Integrating Family Resilience and Family Stress Therapy," *Journal of Marriage and Family*, 2002. 64(May 2002): pp. 349–360.

#253 Speckhard, A., "Inoculating Resilience to Terrorism: Acute and Posttraumatic Stress Responses in U.S. Military, Foreign, and Civilian Services Serving Overseas After September 11th," *Traumatology*, 2002. 8(June): pp. 103–130.

Unit-Level Factors

Positive Command Climate
#31 Castro, C.A., and D. McGurk, "The Intensity of Combat and Behavioral Health Status," *Traumatology*, 2007. 13(4): pp. 6–23.

#148 Brailey, K., et al., "PTSD Symptoms, Life Events, and Unit Cohesion in U.S. Soldiers: Baseline Findings from the Neurocognition Deployment Health Study," *Journal of Traumatic Stress*, 2007. 20(4): pp. 495–503.

#218 Paton, D., "Critical Incident Stress Risk in Police Officers: Managing Resilience and Vulnerability," *Traumatology*, 2006. 12(198): pp. 198–205.

#240 Van Breda, A.D., *Resilience Theory: A Literature Review*. 2001, South African Military Health Service, Military Psychological Institute, Social Work Research & Development: Pretoria, South Africa.

#271 Campbell, D., K. Campbell, and J. Ness, "Resilience Through Leadership," in *Biobehavioral Resilience to Stress*, B.J. Lukey and V. Tepe, Editors. 2008, CRC Press: Boca Raton, FL.

#272 Southwick, S., et al., "Adaptation to Stress and Psychobiological Mechanisms of Resilience," in *Biobehavioral Resilience to Stress*, B.J. Lukey and V. Tepe, Editors. 2008, CRC Press: Boca Raton, FL.

#283 Bliese, P.D., "Social Climates: Drivers of Soldier Well-Being and Resilience," in *Military Life*, C.A. Castro, A.B. Adler, and T. Britt, Editors. 2006, Greenwood Publishing Group: Santa Barbara, CA.

#305 Bartone, P.T., "Hardiness as a Resiliency Resource Under High Stress Conditions," in *Promoting Capabilities to Manage Posttraumatic Stress*, D. Paton, J.M. Violanti, and L.M. Smith, Editors. 2003, Charles C. Thomas Publisher, Ltd.: Springfield, Illinois.

#317 Bowen, G.L., et al., "Promoting the Adaptation of Military Families: An Empirical Test of a Community Practice Model," *Family Relations*, 2003. 52(1): pp. 33–44.

Teamwork
#218 Paton, D., "Critical Incident Stress Risk in Police Officers: Managing Resilience and Vulnerability," *Traumatology*, 2006. 12(198): pp. 198–205.

#351 McCraty, R., et al., "Hew Hope for Correctional Officers: An Innovative Program for Reducing Stress and Health Risks," *Applied Psychophysiology and Biofeedback*, 2009. 34(4).

Cohesion
#45 Eid, J., and B.H. Johnsen, "Acute Stress Reactions After Submarine Accidents," *Military Medicine*, 2002. 167(5): pp. 427–431.

#82 Maguen, S., et al., "Posttraumatic Growth Among Gulf War I Veterans: The Predictive Role of Deployment-Related Experiences and Background Characteristics," *Journal of Loss and Trauma*, 2006. 11(5): pp. 373–388.

148 Brailey, K., et al., "PTSD Symptoms, Life Events, and Unit Cohesion in U.S. Soldiers: Baseline Findings from the Neurocognition Deployment Health Study," *Journal of Traumatic Stress*, 2007. 20(4): pp. 495–503.

218 Paton, D., "Critical Incident Stress Risk in Police Officers: Managing Resilience and Vulnerability," *Traumatology*, 2006. 12(198): pp. 198–205.

340 Adler, A.B., et al., "Battlemind Debriefing and Battlemind Training as Early Interventions with Soldiers Returning from Iraq: Randomized by Platoon," *Journal of Consulting and Clinical Psychology*, 2009. 77(5): pp. 928–940.

Community-Level Factors

Belongingness

13 Vernberg, E.M., et al., "Innovations in Disaster Mental Health: Psychological First Aid," *Professional Psychology: Research and Practice*, 2008. 39(4): pp. 381–388.

23 Bonanno, G.A., et al., "What Predicts Psychological Resilience After Disaster? The Role of Demographics, Resources, and Life Stress," *Journal of Consulting and Clinical Psychology*, 2007. 75(5): pp. 671–682.

51 Friedman, M., and C. Higson-Smith, "Building Psychological Resilience: Learning from the South African Police Service," in *Promoting Capabilities to Manage Posttraumatic Stress: Perspectives on Resilience*, D. Paton, J.M. Violanti, and L.M. Smith, Editors. 2003, Charles C. Thomas Publisher, Ltd.: Springfield, Illinois. pp. 103–118.

60 Hautamaki, A., and P.G. Coleman, "Explanation for Low Prevalence of PTSD Among Older Finnish War Veterans: Social Solidarity and Continued Significance Given to Wartime Sufferings," *Aging and Mental Health*, 2001. 5(2): pp. 165–174.

62 Hoge, E.A., E.D. Austin, and M.H. Pollack, "Resilience: Research Evidence and Conceptual Considerations for Posttraumatic Stress Disorder," *Depression and Anxiety*, 2007. 24(2): pp. 139–152.

66 Johnson, D.M., et al., "Emotional Numbing Weakens Abused Inner-City Women's Resiliency Resources," *Journal of Traumatic Stress*, 2007. 20(2): pp. 197–206.

82 Maguen, S., et al., "Posttraumatic Growth Among Gulf War I Veterans: The Predictive Role of Deployment-Related Experiences and Background Characteristics," *Journal of Loss and Trauma*, 2006. 11(5): pp. 373–388.

101 Qouta, S., et al., "Predictors of Psychological Distress and Positive Resources Among Palestinian Adolescents: Trauma, Child, and Mothering Characteristics," *Child Abuse and Neglect*, 2007. 31(7): pp. 699–717.

152 Black, K., and M. Lobo, "A Conceptual Review of Family Resilience Factors," *Journal of Family Nursing*, 2008. 14(1): pp. 33–55.

178 Conger, R.D., and K.J. Conger, "Resilience in Midwestern Families: Selected Findings from the First Decade of a Prospective, Longitudinal Study," *Journal of Marriage and Family*, 2002. 64(2): pp. 361–373.

183 Tedeschi, R.G., and R.P. Kilmer, "Assessing Strengths, Resilience, and Growth to Guide Clinical Interventions," *Professional Psychology: Research and Practice*, 2005. 36(3): pp. 230–237.

188 Coleman, M., and L. Ganong, "Resilience and Families," *Family Relations*, 2002. 51(2): pp. 101–102.

#193 Lester, P., *Project Focus: Families OverComing Under Stress*. 2008, University of California Los Angeles, National Child Traumatic Stress Network.

#195 Aisenberg, E., and T. Herrenkohl, "Community Violence in Context: Risk and Resilience in Children and Families," *Journal of Interpersonal Violence*, 2008. 23(3): pp. 296–315.

#212 Condly, S.J., "Resilience in Children: A Review of Literature with Implications for Education," *Urban Education*, 2006. 41: pp. 211–236.

#221 Carver, C.S., "Resilience and Thriving: Issues, Models, and Linkages," *Journal of Social Issues*, 1998. 54(2): pp. 245–266.

#226 Hoge, C.W., et al., "Combat Duty in Iraq and Afghanistan, Mental Health Problems, and Barriers to Care," *New England Journal of Medicine*, 2004. 351(1): pp. 13–22.

#229 Tusaie, K., and J. Dyer, "Resilience: A Historical Review of the Construct," *Holist Nurs Pract*, 2004. 18(1): pp. 3–8.

#238 Bonanno, G.A., and A.D. Mancini, "The Human Capacity to Thrive in the Face of Potential Trauma," *Pediatrics*, 2008. 121: pp. 369–375.

#239 Novaco, R.W., T.M. Cook, and I.G. Sarason, "Military Recruit Training: An Arena for Stress-Coping Skills," in *Stress Reduction and Prevention*, D. Meichenbaum and M.E. Jaremko, Editors. 1983, Plenum Press: New York, NY. p. 3.

#240 Van Breda, A.D., *Resilience Theory: A Literature Review*. 2001, South African Military Health Service, Military Psychological Institute, Social Work Research & Development: Pretoria, South Africa.

#241 Norris, F.H., and S.P. Stevens, "Community Resilience and the Principles of Mass Trauma Intervention," *Psychiatry*, 2007. 70(4): pp. 320–328.

#243 O'Donnell, D.A., M.E. Schwab-Stone, and A.Z. Muyeed, "Multidimensional Resilience in Urban Children Exposed to Community Violence," *Child Development*, 2002. 73(4): pp. 1265–1282.

#245 Hobfoll, S.E., et al., "Five Essential Elements of Immediate and Mid-Term Mass Trauma Intervention: Empirical Evidence," *Psychiatry*, 2007. 70(4): pp. 283–315.

#250 Vogt, D.S., and L.R. Tanner, "Risk and Resilience Factors for Posttraumatic Stress Symptomatology in Gulf War I Veterans," *Journal of Traumatic Stress*, 2007. 20(1): pp. 27–38.

#260 King, D.W., et al., "Posttraumatic Stress Disorder in a National Sample of Female and Male Vietnam Veterans: Risk Factors, War Zone Stressors, and Resilience-Recovery Variables," *Journal of Abnormal Psychology*, 1999. 108(1): pp. 164–170.

#273 Friedl, K., and D. Penetar, "Resilience and Survival in Extreme Environments," in *Biobehavioral Resilience to Stress*, B.J. Lukey and V. Tepe, Editors. 2008, CRC Press: Boca Raton, FL

#278 Pfefferbaum, B., et al., "Building Resilience to Mass Trauma Events," in *Handbook on Injury and Violence Prevention*, L.S. Doll, et al., Editors. 2007, Centers for Disease Control and Prevention, National Center for Injury Prevention and Control: Atlanta, GA.

#291 Keane, T.M., et al., "Social Support in Vietnam Veterans with Posttraumatic Stress Disorder: A Comparative Analysis," *Journal of Consulting and Clinical Psychology*, 1985. 53(1): pp. 95–102.

#292 Solomon, Z., M. Mikulincer, and E. Avitzur, "Coping, Locus of Control, Social Support, and Combat-Related Posttraumatic Stress Disorder: A Prospective Study," *Journal of Personality and Social Psychology*, 1988. 55(2): pp. 279–285.

#295 Butler, L.D., L.A. Morland, and G.A. Leskin, "Psychological Resilience in the Face of Terrorism," in *Psychology of Terrorism*, Bonger, et al., Editors. 2007, Oxford University Press: Oxford, UK.

#315 Calhoun, L.G., and R.G. Tedeschi, "Routes to Posttraumatic Growth Through Cognitive Processing," in *Promoting Capabilities to Manage Posttraumatic Stress*, D. Paton, J.M. Violanti, and L.M. Smith, Editors. 2003, Charles C. Thomas Publisher, Ltd.: Springfield, Illinois.

#317 Bowen, G.L., et al., "Promoting the Adaptation of Military Families: An Empirical Test of a Community Practice Model," *Family Relations*, 2003. 52(1): pp. 33–44.

Cohesion

#20 Benedek, D.M., and E.C. Ritchie, "'Just-in-Time' Mental Health Training and Surveillance for the Project HOPE Mission," *Military Medicine*, 2006. 171(10 Suppl 1): pp. 63–65.

#169 Nucifora, F., et al., *Building Resistance, Resilience, and Recovery in the Wake of School and Workplace Violence*. 2007, Department of Psychiatry and Behavioral Health Sciences, Johns Hopkins University School of Medicine.

#252 Maguire, B., and P. Hagan, "Disasters and Communities: Understanding Social Resilience," *Australian Journal of Emergency Management*, 2007. 22(2): pp. 16–20.

#280 Lepore, S., and T. Revenson, "Relationships Between Posttraumatic Growth and Resilience: Recovery, Resistance, and Reconfiguration," in *Handbook of Posttraumatic Growth: Research and Practice*, L.G. Calhoun and R.G. Tedeschi, Editors. 2006, Lawrence Erlbaum Associates: Mahwah, NJ.

Connectedness

#3 Vernberg, E.M., et al., "Innovations in Disaster Mental Health: Psychological First Aid," *Professional Psychology: Research and Practice*, 2008. 39(4): pp. 381–388.

#164 Walsh, F., "Family Resilience: A Framework for Clinical Practice," *Family Process*, 2003. 42(1).

#195 Aisenberg, E., and T. Herrenkohl, "Community Violence in Context: Risk and Resilience in Children and Families," *Journal of Interpersonal Violence*, 2008. 23(3): pp. 296–315.

#245 Hobfoll, S.E., et al., "Five Essential Elements of Immediate and Mid-Term Mass Trauma Intervention: Empirical Evidence," *Psychiatry*, 2007. 70(4): pp. 283–315.

#275 Rohall, D., and J. Martin, "The Impact of Social Structural Conditions on Psychological Resilience to Stress," in *Biobehavioral Resilience to Stress.*, B.J. Lukey and V. Tepe, Editors. 2008, CRC Press: Boca Raton, FL.

#278 Pfefferbaum, B., et al., "Building Resilience to Mass Trauma Events," in *Handbook on Injury and Violence Prevention*, L.S. Doll, et al., Editors. 2007, Centers for Disease Control and Prevention, National Center for Injury Prevention and Control: Atlanta, GA.

#318 Bell, C.C., "Cultivating Resiliency in Youth," *Journal of Adolescent Health*, 2001. 29: pp. 375–381.

Collective Efficacy

#245 Hobfoll, S.E., et al., "Five Essential Elements of Immediate and Mid-Term Mass Trauma Intervention: Empirical Evidence," *Psychiatry*, 2007. 70(4): pp. 283–315.

#252 Maguire, B., and P. Hagan, "Disasters and Communities: Understanding Social Resilience," *Australian Journal of Emergency Management*, 2007. 22(2): pp. 16–20.

#268 Bliese, P.D., and C.A. Castro, "The Soldier Adaptation Model (SAM): Applications to Peacekeeping Research," in *The Psychology of the Peacekeeper: Lessons from the Field*, T. Britt and A.B. Adler, Editors. 2003, Praeger: Westport, Connecticut.

Full List of Resilience Programs

Table C.1
Resilience Programs (n=77)

Program	Resilience Content	Target Audience	Sponsor/ Funding
Army Center for Enhanced Performance (ACEP)	Mental, physical	Primarily soldiers, also family and Department of the Army civilians	Army
Adaptive Disclosure Training	Social	Service members	Marine Corps
Assessment and Treatment of Wounded Warrior's Families	Social	Families	Navy and Marine Corps
Battlemind (now called Resiliency Training)	Mental, physical	Soldiers, their spouses, and leaders	Army
Bowling Green State University (BGSU) Spiritual Resilience Program	Spiritual	College students	BGSU
Bootcamp Survival Training for Navy Recruits—A Prescription (BOOTSTRAP)	Mental, social	Navy recruits	Navy
Bullet-Proofing the Mind	Mental	Service members and leaders	Department of Defense
Caregiver Occupational Stress Control	Mental, social	Medical caregivers	Navy
Center for Mind Body Medicine	Mental, physical, spiritual	Health professionals and individuals exposed to stress	Civilian
Center of Spiritual Leadership	Spiritual	Service members	Army
Center for the Study of Traumatic Stress	Mental	Health care providers, service members, and their families	DCoE
Combat Operational Stress First Aid (COSFA)	Mental, social	Service members and caregivers	Navy and Marine Corps
The Coming Home Project	Mental, physical, spiritual	Service members, their families, and providers	Civilian

Table C.1—Continued

Program	Resilience Content	Target Audience	Sponsor/ Funding
Community Capacity Building for Military Families	Mental, social	Military families	Civilian
Community Stress Prevention Center	Mental, physical, social, spiritual	Individuals exposed to high stress	Civilian (Israel)
Compassion Fatigue Process Improvement Project	Social	Military health care providers	Army
Comprehensive COSC Training	Mental, physical, social, spiritual	Military members, their families and leaders, and medical and religious professionals	Navy and Marine Corps
Comprehensive Soldier Fitness (CSF) program	Mental, physical, social, spiritual	Soldiers, their families, and Army civilians	Army
Corporate Athlete/Full Engagement/Energy Management	Mental, physical, social, spiritual	Leaders	Civilian, private sector
Deployment Safety and Resiliency Team (DSRT)	Mental, social	Centers for Disease Control and Prevention deployment teams	Centers for Disease Control and Prevention
Employee Engagement Program (NSA)	Mental, physical, social, spiritual[a]	Leaders primarily, as well as general workforce	Internal executive champions provide funding. Private sector materials are purchased.
The Energy Project	Mental, physical, social, spiritual	Organizations and individuals, senior executives and corporate employees	Civilian, private sector
Families OverComing Under Stress (FOCUS)	Mental, social	Military families with children	Navy and Marine Corps
The Family Check-Up	Mental, social	Families	Civilian
Family Optimization Systems (Magis Group; FAMOPS)	Mental, physical	Military family members	Civilian, private sector
Fort Bliss Restoration and Resilience Center	Mental, social	Soldiers who have endured combat stress	Department of Defense
Gallup Consulting	Mental	Individuals and groups	Civilian, private sector
Health and Wellness Promotion Program	Mental, physical	Service members, their families, and leaders	Navy

Table C.1—Continued

Program	Resilience Content	Target Audience	Sponsor/Funding
HeartMath	Mental, physical	Individuals exposed to high stress	Institute of HeartMath (nonprofit research and educational charter) and HeartMath LLC
Human Systems Optimization (HSO)	Mental, physical	Individuals and organizations	Civilian, private sector
(Mental Health and Operational Stress Injury) Joint Speakers Bureau (JSB)	Mental, social	Service members, leaders, and families	Department of National Defence, Canada
Kansas Air National Guard Resilience program	Mental, social, spiritual	Guardsmen, their families, and leaders	National Guard
Landing Gear	Mental, physical, spiritual	Airmen, their families, and leaders	Air Force
Life Skills Training	Social	Service members and their families	Civilian
Marine Resilience Study (MRS)	Mental, physical, social	Marines	VA, Navy, and Marine Corps
Martial Arts Center of Excellence (MACE)	Mental, physical, spiritual	Marines	Marine Corps
Mental Toughness for Operations	Mental	Service members	Australian Defence Force
Mindfulness-based Mind Fitness Training (MMFT)	Mental, physical, social, spiritual	Military service members	Kluge Foundation, DCoE, and Army
National Guard Resiliency Program	Mental, social, spiritual	Guardsmen, their families, and leaders	National Guard
Navy Special Warfare (NSW) Resilience Enterprise	Social	NSW operators and their families	Navy
One Shot . . . One Kill (OSOK)	Not available	Service members	Air Force
Operational Stress Control and Readiness (OSCAR)	Mental, physical	Military members and leaders	Marine Corps

Table C.1—Continued

Program	Resilience Content	Target Audience	Sponsor/ Funding
Operational Stress Injury Social Support (OSISS)	Social	Military members and families (including bereaved families)	Department of National Defence and Veterans Affairs Canada
Our Strength in Families (OSiF)	Mental, social	Military couples and families	Civilian
Passport Toward Success	Mental, social	Children, adolescents, and families in the Indiana National Guard	Purdue University and Indiana National Guard
The Penn Resiliency Project (PRP)/ Master Resilience Training (MRT)	Mental, social	Youth, young adults, students, executives, leaders, military service members, and their families	PRP: National Institute of Mental Health. MRT: Army.
Positive Psychology for Youth Project	Mental, social	High school students	Department of Education
Preventive Psychological Health Demonstration Project (PPHDP)	Mental, physical	Active-duty service members and family members	Department of Defense
Promoting Alternative THinking Strategies (PATHS)	Mental, social	Elementary-aged children, their educators, and counselors	Program is purchased by a school or community agency
Project Armor	Mental, social	Adolescents from military families, typically middle-school students	Department of Defense
Provider Resiliency Training (PRT)	Social	Military health care providers	Army
Ready Good to Go	Not available	Service members	Department of Defense
Real Warriors Campaign	Mental	Service members, families, leaders, and caregivers	DCoE
Returning Warrior Workshops	Social	Sailors returning from mobilization or deployment and a family member	Department of Defense
School Mental Health Team (SMHT)	Mental, social	Youth, parents, and staff at schools in military communities	Congress (through PTSD/TBI/BH funding)
Senior Leader Wellness Enhancement Seminar (SLWES)	Social	Senior military leaders and their spouses	Army

Table C.1—Continued

Program	Resilience Content	Target Audience	Sponsor/ Funding
Sesame Workshop	Social	Children	DCoE
Soldier Evaluation for Life Fitness (SELF)	Mental, physical, spiritual	Soldiers	Army
Soldier Wellness Assessment Program (SWAP)	Mental, physical, spiritual	Service members	Army
Strategic Outreach to Families of All Reservists (SOFAR)	Mental, social	Families of Reservists and National Guard	National Guard and Reserve Components
Spiritual Fitness Center	Spiritual	Service members and their families	Navy
Spiritual Leadership Theory	Spiritual	Leaders	Civilian
Spiritual Reintegration and Resiliency Training (SRRT)	Spiritual	Service members, their families, and leaders	Army
Spiritual Warrior Training Program	Mental, spiritual	Soldiers in basic combat training, especially those identified as high-risk	Army
Stoic Resilience Training	Mental	Service members	Army
Syntrak International	Social	Service members	Civilian
Trauma Risk Management System (TRiM)	Mental	Service members, health care providers	British Armed Forces
Warrior Adventure Quest (WAQ)	Mental, physical	Service members	Army
Warrior Mind Training	Mental	Service members	Department of Defense
Warrior Optimization Systems (WAROPS)	Mental	Service members	Civilian, private sector
Warrior Resilience Coaching	Mental	Service members	Not available
Warrior Resilience Program (Ft. Hood)	Mental, physical	Military members and their families	Army
Warrior Resilience and Thriving (WRT)	Mental, spiritual	Military members and their families	No formal funding
Warrior Resiliency Program (WRP)	Mental, physical	Service members, their families, leaders, and community	Army
Warrior Transition Briefs	Social	Service members	Marine Corps

Table C.1—Continued

Program	Resilience Content	Target Audience	Sponsor/ Funding
Warrior Wellness Innovation Network (WWIN) Wellness Program	Mental, physical	Service members	Department of Defense
Yellow Ribbon Reintegration Program	Mental, physical, spiritual	Service members and their families	Army

[a] Program representatives specified that this program also contains emotional content.

Brief Program Descriptions

Table D.1
Army Center for Enhanced Performance

Feature	Description
Website/online documentation	http://www.acep.army.mil/
Concept	Psychological training strengthens the mind-body connection and enhances human performance. Key components of training are (1) mental skills foundations, (2) building confidence, (3) goal setting, (4) attention control, (5) energy management, and (6) integrating imagery. This program draws from applied sport, health, and social psychology.
Mission	To develop the full potential of soldiers and families using a systematic educational and developmental process grounded in cutting edge performance psychology and learning strategies in order to enhance adaptive thinking, mental agility, and self-regulation skills essential to the pursuit of overall personal strength, professional excellence, and the Warrior Ethos across the Army.
Background	ACEP originated from the Center for Enhanced Performance at the U.S. Military Academy at West Point, N.Y., which has trained soldiers since 1993. ACEP is one of three programs that will be integrated into the Army's CSF program.
Resilience content	Mental, physical
Target audience	Primarily soldiers. Also family and Department of the Army (DA) civilians.
Phases of military deployment addressed	Primarily predeployment. Some in theater and post-deployment.
Services	(1) Mental skills education and biofeedback training for individuals and groups. (2) Unit predeployment and team-building training workshops. (3) Warfare language and culture courses. (4) Kinesthetic Room training that uses high-tech simulations to sharpen soldiers' skills. (5) Executive leader seminars to advance managerial proficiency for senior leaders. (6) Family readiness programs (currently pilot programs) to inspire personal and family growth. (7) Warrior transition programs to promote successful transition from injury back to duty or civilian life. (8) A Learning and Teaching Program (LTP) for developing intellectual self-awareness and self-regulation.

Table D.1—Continued

Feature	Description
Mode of delivery and dose	Workshops with 20 to 100 participants (typically between 40 and 60), 6 to 8 hours long. LTP includes 8 to 12 hours of training and an additional 8 to 12 hours of exercises. Individual mastery sessions are voluntary and available for walk-ins. 300–400 of these were held across all 9 sites during the summer of 2009.
Location of services	ACEP headquarters in West Point, N.Y. Sites in (1) Ft. Bragg, N.C.; (2) Ft. Jackson, S.C; (3) Walter Reed Medical Center, Washington, D.C.; (4) Ft. Lewis, Wash.; (5) Ft. Sam Houston, Tex.; (6) Ft. Gordon, Ga.; (7) Ft. Hood, Tex.; (8) Ft. Knox, Ky.; (9) Ft. Bliss, Tex.
Staff	Across all locations: 11 PhDs and 27 MAs in sports, performance, and clinical psychology. At each location: one site manager, 3 to 10 Performance Enhancement Specialists (PES), and support staff.
Training requirements of staff	Four-week certification at ACEP headquarters in West Point and certification by Association of Applied Sport Psychology.
Client details	Soldiers: Walter Reed (primary client), Training and Doctrine Command (TRADOC), Forces Command (FORSCOM), U.S. Army Special Operations Command (USASOC), Medical Command (MEDCOM), Special Operations, Stryker Brigade Combat Teams (SBCTs), Terminal High-Altitude Area Defense (THAAD), Drill Sergeant School, and other army schools. During the summer of 2009, 300 to 400 soldiers attended individual mastery sessions. Services are provided to families of soldiers at Ft. Lewis and Ft. Bliss and to Department of the Army civilians at Ft. Gordon.
Sponsor/funding	Army

Table D.2
Battlemind (now called Resiliency Training)

Feature	Description
Website/online documentation	https://www.battlemind.army.mil/
Concept	A comprehensive mental health training program designed to prepare service members for the demands and challenges of military life, combat, and transitioning home. Battlemind is defined as the warrior's inner strength to face the environment with courage, confidence, and resilience. This program draws from positive psychology, cognitive restructuring, mindfulness, and research on posttraumatic stress, unit cohesion, occupational health models, organizational leadership, and deployment.
Mission	To prepare soldiers mentally for the rigors of deployment and combat, to assist soldiers in successful transition back home, to prepare soldiers to assist a "battle buddy" during deployment and transition home, and to prepare soldiers for possible redeployment.
Background	The U.S. Army's first validated mental health training program, developed by WRAIR and based on data from the Land Combat Study and others. Mandated Army-wide in 2007. This program is now being integrated into the Army's CSF program as a component of Resilience Training.
Resilience content	Mental, physical
Target audience	Soldiers, their spouses, and leaders
Phases of military deployment addressed	Predeployment, in theater, and post-deployment
Services	Integrated series of life cycle and deployment cycle training modules/classes. (1) Life cycle training includes Battlemind Warrior Resiliency, which teaches soldiers to identify peers at risk for psychological trauma. (2) Deployment cycle training is provided for soldiers and their spouses in preparation for all deployment transitions. (3) Soldier-support training captures populations and subjects that life cycle and deployment cycle modules do not (e.g., National Guard and Reserve Component–specific issues). (4) Specified training is available for medical personnel. (5) A Train-the-Trainer program is available for military Chaplains (BMT3C, a five-day program).
Mode of delivery and dose	Course modules are typically one to three hours of instruction and discussion. These occur primarily in platoon-sized classes. For some groups, such as health care providers, class sizes are much smaller. A Master Resilience Trainer course includes about 150 service members and involves discussion, interactive techniques, and role-playing. Online resources are also available.
Location of services	Army-wide
Staff	Master Resilience Trainers, TRADOC staff; Battalion Aid Station (BAS). Some modules are delivered by Brigade Mental Health and COSC teams.
Training requirements of staff	Training materials developed by WRAIR and the Soldier and Family Support Branch, U.S. Army Medical Department Center and School (AMEDDC&S).
Client details	Not available
Sponsor/funding	Army

Table D.3
Combat Operational Stress Control Program/Operational Stress Control and Readiness

Feature	Description
Website/online documentation	http://www.usmc-mccs.org/cosc/
Concept	COSC encompasses all Marine Corps (MC) policies and programs designed to prevent, identify, and holistically treat mental injuries caused by combat or other military operations. The COSC model is unit leader–oriented, multidisciplinary, integrated throughout the organization, without stigma, consistent with the Warrior Ethos, and focused on wellness, prevention, and resilience. OSCAR, a COSC program, creates a two-way bridge between operational and mental health cultures by embedding mental health providers at the level of infantry regiments.
Mission	To create and preserve a ready force and to promote the long-term health and well-being of individual Marines, sailors, and family members. To support commander and service members' psychological health through consultation, training, prevention, monitoring, early intervention, and clinical mental health services capabilities.
Background	The current COSC model was developed in 2007 by a working group of Marine leaders, chaplains, and medical and mental health professionals. OSCAR began in 1999, in the 2nd Marine Division at Camp Lejeune, N.C., and expanded to include other Marine divisions in 2003. In 2007, the DoD announced other mental health programs that will be also be based on this model.
Resilience content	Mental, physical, social, spiritual
Target audience	Military members, family members, leaders, and medical and religious professionals
Phases of military deployment addressed	Predeployment, in theater, and post-deployment
Services	Marines receive COSC training in each career school and for any deployment over 90 days. COSC training for military leaders emphasizes five core leader functions: to strengthen (e.g., promote stress inoculation, coping skills, and social cohesion), to mitigate (i.e., to prevent stress injuries through monitoring and alleviating stressors), to identify at-risk individuals, to treat (e.g., by self-aid, peer support, or direction to mental health professionals), and to reintegrate those with stress injuries back to full duty. Other COSC programs, such as the FOCUS Project, provide education and skills training for military families. OSCAR staff provides mental health support and command consultation to help leaders build individual and unit strength, resilience, and readiness. OSCAR staff is also integrated with military members to provide early interventions or treatment when appropriate.
Mode of delivery and dose	Most COSC training occurs in classrooms. For any Marine deployment over 90 days, training occurs within 60 days of deployment, again within 60 days of departure from theater, and then again between 60 to 120 days after return. OSCAR staff members are embedded within military units in training and in theater.
Location of services	Across the Marine Corps and Navy in operational settings and on base.

Table D.3—Continued

Feature	Description
Staff	COSC core staff members are drawn from Headquarters MC departments, Marine Corps Combat Development Command, operational commands, the Navy Bureau of Medicine and Surgery, the Navy chaplaincy, the Veterans Administration, the National Center for PTSD, and many other educational and research organizations. Within each regiment's unit, an OSCAR mental health team comprises one mental health provider (psychiatrist, psychologist, social worker, or clinical nurse specialist), one or more extenders (psychiatric technician corpsman, other medical service providers, chaplains, etc.), senior mentors (executive officers and senior enlisted advisors), and peer mentors (selected officers and enlisted Marines).
Training requirements of staff	Among COSC programs, staff training is specific to the service delivered. OSCAR staff training is provided via Marine Corps Headquarters. Peer mentors, senior mentors, and previously deployed extenders require four half-days of specialized training. Mental health staff and new extenders require five half-days.
Client details	Not available
Sponsor/funding	MC and DoD

Table D.4
Employee Engagement Program, National Security Agency

Feature	Description
Website/online documentation	http://www.dcoe.health.mil/DCoEV2/Content/navigation/documents pdf-2009%2011%2009/2009%2011%2003_1120-1135_rac_pille.pdf
Concept	Becoming fully engaged requires managing energy, not time, to sustain high performance. This program is grounded in performance psychology, exercise physiology, and nutrition. The conceptual model for this program is a pyramid with four key areas, beginning with physical at the base and moving up to emotional, mental, and spiritual as crucial energy-management skills.
Mission	To strategically train leaders to increase their capacity for performing under pressure and to improve their ability to expend and recover energy more efficiently and effectively.
Background	Loehr and Groppel's Human Performance Institute (HPI) Corporate Athlete Program was adapted by NSA health professionals for use within DoD. The DoD version was called Employee Engagement Program and was implemented by the NSA in October 2005. Based on feedback from military members assigned to NSA, the program name will be changed to Full Engagement Program, which sounds more inclusive.
Resilience content	Mental, physical, social, spiritual
Target audience	Primarily leaders. Condensed versions are available for the general workforce.
Phases of military deployment addressed	Not applicable
Services	(1) Pretest biometrics and health risk assessments. (2) Group discussions of the four dimensions of energy: physical, emotional, mental, and spiritual. (3) Creation of individualized action plans based on personal data, goals, and concepts and principles learned in class.
Mode of delivery and dose	The program is delivered in classrooms. Workshop length is 2.5 days for leaders and four or eight hours for the general workforce. (Clients return for post-program evaluations after 6 months.) Workbook and reference materials are purchased from HPI. An online course is currently in development.
Location of services	Washington, D.C., and also at satellite organizations worldwide.
Staff	The Employee Engagement Program is taught by a core staff team of one psychologist, one fitness expert, one applied behavioral scientist, and one nurse.
Training requirements of staff	First instructors attended HPI's train-the-trainer program. Then, each new trainer participates in the 2.5-day version of the program and is coached when first on the teaching platform.
Client details	Variations of the Corporate Athlete Program have been also been used by GlaxcoSmithKline, Dell, Proctor and Gamble, Southwest Airlines, Pepsi, Estee Lauder, and Smith Barney.
Sponsor/funding	Internal executive champions provide funding. Private sector materials are purchased.

Table D.5
The Energy Project

Feature	Description
Website/online documentation	http://www.theenergyproject.com/
Concept	Becoming fully engaged requires managing energy, not time, to sustain high performance. This program is grounded in performance psychology, exercise physiology, and nutrition. The conceptual model for this program is a pyramid with four key areas, beginning with physical at the base and moving up to emotional, mental, and spiritual as crucial energy-management skills.
Mission	To strategically train leaders to increase their capacity for performing under pressure and to improve their ability to expend and recover energy more efficiently and effectively.
Background	Founded in 2003 by Tony Schwartz. Based on the program by LGE Performance Systems, now called the Human Performance Institute (HPI), which trains individuals, primarily athletes, to improve physical performance by better managing energy across four dimensions: (1) physical, (2) emotional, (3) mental, and (4) spiritual. Schwartz helped LGE extend the program to executives and business people, creating the Corporate Athlete Program with Loehr. Schwarz then created the Energy Project to focus on the latter three dimensions.
Resilience content	Mental, physical, social, spiritual
Target audience	Organizations and individuals. Senior executives and corporate employees.
Phases of military deployment addressed	Not applicable
Services	(1) The Firing on All Cylinders program comprises half-day modules on each of these energy dimensions: physical, emotional, mental, and spiritual. Participants gain increased awareness of the costs and benefits of current behaviors. Sessions are interactive, experiential, and focused on actionable strategies. Participants learn and practice positive rituals (i.e., highly specific energy-management strategies). (2) Ritual Coaching provides individualized coaching between modules. (3) Renewal-in-Action extends the Firing on All Cylinders program by providing additional focus on physical energy (e.g., nutrition and fitness). (4) Organizational Energy Audits (OEA) are conducted to identify and quantify organizations' current practices. (5) Keynote presentations are provided. (6) A train-the-trainer program is available for the Firing on All Cylinders curriculum.
Mode of delivery and dose	Mostly in-person small group discussions, with 15 to 30 participants. Also larger presentations. Some services are provided by phone and webinars. The full program is 16 hours: four hours for each of four modules. Ideally, one module is presented per month. Clients can also receive abbreviated versions of the full program (e.g., the course has been presented in half a day).
Location of services	Services are provided on site.
Staff	Six to seven facilitators and/or coaches in the U.S. and the same number in Europe. Additional independent contractors are brought on for larger projects.

Table D.5—Continued

Feature	Description
Training requirements of staff	Energy Project trainers require extensive facilitation experience and one to five years of employment experience at the Energy Project.
Client details	Corporate and organizational clients include Sony Pictures Entertainment, Ernst & Young, Google, Kaiser Permanente, Deloitte Touche, and Citibank. Public and private sector clients include the Cleveland Clinic, the Los Angeles Police Department, and Save the Children.
Sponsor/funding	Private sector

**Table D.6
Gallup Consulting**

Feature	Description
Website/online documentation	http://www.gallup.com/home.aspx
Concept	Performance outcomes are improved by focusing on both individual and organizational levels. For each level, research-based tools can be administered that combine engagement, strengths, and well-being in meaningful and actionable ways.
Mission	To evaluate a client's strategy, then help the organization's leaders devise effective approaches to build employees' and customers' emotional engagement.
Background	The Gallup Organization was founded by George Gallup in 1935 and was originally called the American Institute of Public Opinion. Today, Gallup provides services worldwide in public opinion polling, market research, and management and leadership consulting.
Resilience content	Mental
Target audience	Individuals and groups
Phases of military deployment addressed	Not applicable
Services	(1) StrengthsFinder: An online measure of personal talent that identifies areas where an individual's greatest potential for building strengths exist. (2) Well-Being Tracker: Tools to assess individual well-being across career, social, financial, physical, and community dimensions. (3) Q-12 and Adult Trait Hope instruments: Tools to assess employee engagement and hope levels.
Mode of delivery and dose	Online resources include personal journals, discussion forums, and development activities. The Gallup team often provides consultation via weekly phone sessions with clients.
Location of services	Gallup has offices in 14 U.S. city centers and 26 cities overseas.
Staff	More than 2,500 employees, including Masters- and PhD-level market researchers, evaluators, methodologists, statisticians, sociologists, and psychologists.
Training requirements of staff	Not applicable
Client details	Federal agencies, state governments, Fortune 500 companies, and nonprofit organizations
Sponsor/funding	Private

Table D.7
HeartMath

Feature	Description
Website/online documentation	http://www.heartmath.org/
Concept	Research-based tools and technologies increase people's ability to self-regulate and improve resilience.
Mission	To help establish heart-based living and global coherence by inspiring people to connect with the intelligence and guidance of their own hearts.
Background	Founded in 1991 and adapted for the military in 2007. HeartMath is credited with first identifying the physiological state of coherence (or resonance) as an optimal state of emotional, cognitive, and physical functioning.
Resilience content	Mental, physical
Target audience	Individuals exposed to high stress
Phases of military deployment addressed	Predeployment, in theater, and post-deployment
Services	For military members, predeployment resiliency and post-deployment/reintegration training workshops. Topics covered include identifying causes of stress and energy drain and achieving coherent physical and mental states in challenging situations. (1) Self-regulation is practiced and improved using technology that measures heart rate variability and provides audio and visual feedback. (2) Emotional resilience training is provided one-on-one by phone. (3) Peer mentoring is available for active-duty service members, veterans, and military family members.
Mode of delivery and dose	Online audio and video presentations, teleseminars, and in-person workshops. Program workshop duration ranges from two hours to three days. One-on-one programs are typically delivered in four to six 30- to 60-minute phone sessions.
Location of services	HeartMath program tools are currently employed by clinicians in over 50 military and VA hospitals and medical centers, including Walter Reed, Mayo, Duke, Stanford, the University of California, San Francisco (UCSF), and the University of North Carolina (UNC).
Staff	For military members, the program management team includes researchers, military advisors from all branches, and a content development team. Program providers include veteran credentialed providers, credentialed mental health providers, credentialed HeartMath providers, HeartMath staff trainers, and certified military instructors

Table D.7—Continued

Feature	Description
Training requirements of staff	(1) Master training for professionals previously trained by the Institute of HeartMath or HeartMath LLC, who have substantial experience conducting HeartMath Resiliency Train-the-Trainer programs. (2) The Train-the-Trainer program is an intensive three- to –five-day certification training including a teach-back component. (3) One-on-one Providers Certification is a prerequisite course for individuals who want to be providers and enroll in the Train-the-Trainer program. (4) The HeartMath Interventions Program is available for training credentialed mental health and health care professionals.
Client details	HeartMath programs have been developed for police, firefighters, nurses, educators, corporate management and staff, and military populations, including the Navy, Kansas National Guard, South Dakota National Guard, and DoD.
Sponsor/funding	Institute of HeartMath (a nonprofit research and educational charter) and HeartMath LLC

Table D.8
Joint Speakers Bureau

Feature	Description
Website/online documentation	http://www.cmp-cpm.forces.gc.ca/cen/ps/mho-smb/jsb-bso-eng.asp
Concept	A systematic mental health education campaign to reach the military population at every level of development. The program is developed and delivered by military members who have recovered from a mental health condition (i.e., peers), military family members, and mental health clinicians.
Mission	To develop, deliver, and evaluate the mental health education of Canadian Forces (CF) members and families. To reduce stigma and change attitudes and behaviors for those with mental health problems.
Background	JSB was initiated in 2007. The program was previously subsumed under OSISS peer support (see below) but was expanded to include a focus on mental health education and illness prevention.
Resilience content	Mental, social
Target audience	Service members, leaders, and families
Phases of military deployment addressed	Predeployment, in theater, and post-deployment
Services	(1) Educational campaigns to inform individual soldiers about mental health issues. (2) Integrated leadership training to help leaders foster group cohesion and unit morale. Also teaches leaders supportive intervention skills to be used in collaboration with health service resources. (3) Basic military qualification courses to improve service members' mental health literacy (e.g., ability to identify unhelpful coping strategies), stigma reduction, and skill development (e.g., developing successful coping strategies). Classroom interactions teach military personnel concrete actions to deal with stress. (4) Professional development lectures tailored for specific audiences (e.g., military units, chaplains, CF case managers). (5) Family curriculum teaches coping, communication, reintegration, and parenting skills.
Mode of delivery and dose	Curriculum is delivered in person by peers and mental health professionals. Speakers are chosen to match audience needs. Courses range from 3 to 8.5 hours in duration. As of June 2009, predeployment training for military members and their families involves 16 hours of participation.
Location of services	Canada
Staff	Management teams include mental health experts, advisors, mental health professionals, and former or active CF members and their families.
Training requirements of staff	After a rigorous screening and selection process, mental health professionals and peer candidates are required to participate in a two-week training course.
Client details	Not available
Sponsor/funding	Department of National Defence, Canada

Table D.9
Landing Gear

Feature	Description
Website/online documentation	http://airforcemedicine.afms.mil/idc/groups/public/documents/ webcontent/knowledgejunction.hcst?functionalarea=AFSuicidePreve ntionPrgm&doctype=subpage&docname=CTB_095710&incbanner=0
Concept	A standardized approach to mental illness prevention and mental health education. Based on the metaphor that, no matter how powerful an aircraft is, properly functioning landing gear is necessary to safely launch and recover. Effective risk recognition and help-seeking behavior are the functional equivalent of landing gear for Airmen.
Mission	To increase the recognition of Airmen suffering from traumatic stress symptoms and connect them with helping resources.
Background	Program released in April 2008
Resilience content	Mental, physical, spiritual
Target audience	Airmen, their families, and leaders
Phases of military deployment addressed	Primarily pre- and post-deployment. Some mental health support is provided in theater.
Services	(1) Predeployment classes address deployment stress, the deployed environment, typical reactions, mental illness prevention, and getting help. (2) Post-deployment classes emphasize typical reactions, reintegration and reunion, and getting help. (3) Specific training is provided for redeployment preparation and addresses Airmen's spiritual, medical, mental health, financial, legal, child care, and administrative needs.
Mode of delivery and dose	In-person briefings range from 15 minutes to one hour in duration. Typically one-time-only classes, but can also be recurring.
Location of services	The program is provided at existing training events, such as the annual Mental Health conference.
Staff	Mental health personnel
Training requirements of staff	Curriculum is provided for speakers. No additional training required.
Client details	Not available
Sponsor/funding	Air Force

Table D.10
Marine Resiliency Study

Feature	Description
Website/online documentation	http://www.usmc-mccs.org/cosc/conf2007/documents/3A%20 1Posttraumatic%20Stress%20Disorder%20MRS%20Talk%20Baker. pdf
Concept	A prospective longitudinal study of Marines' risk and resilience for combat stress injuries and stress illnesses (especially PTSD). The range of factors considered includes genetic and biological, psychological and past history, social (unit and family), and environmental (stress exposures).
Mission	To learn how the Marine Corps can mitigate preexisting risk and prevent, identify, and treat operational and combat stress injuries.
Background	This study was initiated in July 2008. The research team is multidisciplinary. MRS is the first prospective study to examine trajectories of adaptation to combat.
Resilience content	Mental, physical, social
Target audience	Marines
Phases of military deployment addressed	Data are collected pre- and post-deployment.
Services	To date, data have been collected from 1,600 Marines. In total, 2,300–2,400 will be invited to participate. Data are gathered within month prior to deployment and then at one week, three months, and six months post-deployment. The primary outcome variable is assessed using the Clinician-Administered PTSD Scale (CAPS). Predictors of interest include early childhood trauma, general intelligence, psychosocial support, and genetic and neurobiological resilience and risk factors.
Mode of delivery and dose	Not applicable
Location of services	Marines are evaluated at Camp Pendleton and MCAGCC 29 Palms, Calif.
Staff	Not applicable
Training requirements of staff	Not applicable
Client details	Not applicable
Sponsor/funding	Veterans Affairs, Marine Corps, and Navy Medicine

Table D.11
Mindfulness-Based Mind Fitness Training

Feature	Description
Website/online documentation	https://digitalndulibrary.ndu.edu/u?/ndupress,39443 For general information: info@mind-fitness-training.org
Concept	Mind fitness is improved with attention and concentration exercises that change the brain structurally and functionally. This course emphasizes mental agility, emotional regulation, attention, working memory, and situational awareness.
Mission	To protect soldiers as they prepare for deployment and experience stressors. To improve mission performance and reduce rates of PTSD, depression, and anxiety in soldiers upon return.
Background	MMFT is based on a well-established course (Mindfulness-Based Stress Reduction) that has been shown to improve attentional functioning and reduce the negative effects of stress. MMFT was tailored specifically for military predeployment. In 2008, a pilot study followed 35 Marines who received MMFT before deploying to Iraq. Upcoming studies will compare the effectiveness of MMFT with Battlemind and determine optimal dosing of MMFT.
Resilience content	Mental, physical, social, spiritual
Target audience	Service members
Phases of military deployment addressed	Predeployment
Services	The MMFT course teaches mindfulness (attention control and concentration), stress resilience skills (to recognize and cope with physiological and psychological stress), and applications to counterinsurgency environment. Exercises are to be practiced at least 30 minutes per day during training.
Mode of delivery and dose	MMFT is provided to groups of 20 to 25 participants at a time. The course involved 24 hours of curriculum taught over eight weeks. One 15-minute individual interview is provided in Week 3.
Location of services	On-site at organizations, anywhere in the United States.
Staff	Curricula for new trainers is currently being developed.
Training requirements of staff	Not available
Client details	Military service members, law enforcement officers, intelligence analysts and agents, firefighters, emergency responders, disaster relief and crisis workers, and care providers.
Sponsor/funding	The MMFT pilot study (2008) was funded by the Kluge Foundation and DCoE. Army has funded upcoming studies. It is a 501(c)(3) nonprofit research and training organization.

Table D.12
National Guard Resiliency Program

Feature	Description
Website/online documentation	http://www.kansas.gov/ksadjutantgeneral/Library/Resiliency/Resiliency%20home.htm
Concept	Tools and techniques can be provided in advance of life's challenges. Program is rooted in cognitive-behavioral therapy.
Mission	To further strengthen National Guard members and their families to better handle life's challenges.
Background	Program was initiated in Kansas in 2008 and is referred to as the Kansas Adjutant General's Department Resiliency Center. The program was expanded to other states in 2009. It incorporates training developed by the Israeli military and NATO.
Resilience content	Mental, social, spiritual
Target audience	Guardsmen, their families, and leaders
Phases of military deployment addressed	Predeployment and in theater
Services	(1) WarFighter Diaries Program: A social networking website where service members and families can retrieve and present information about their experiences, challenges, and resources. Downloadable 3- to 5-minute videos of soldiers' accounts of their own experiences are available. (2) Flashforward Program: Curriculum delivered via lectures, videos, and small group discussions. Four blocks of discussion are focused on leadership, one block on spiritual issues (religiosity), and one block on family and reintegration issues.
Mode of delivery and dose	Lectures, small group discussions, videos, information websites, and social networking websites. The Flashforward Program is delivered to groups of 40 to 45 participants and is eight hours in duration.
Location of services	Kansas, Connecticut, Hawaii, Michigan, New Jersey, North Carolina, and Pennsylvania
Staff	The Flashforward Program is taught by teams of three previously deployed service members, one chaplain or chaplain's assistant, and one family support coordinator or director of psychological health.
Training requirements of staff	A two-day Train-the-Trainer program is required for Flashforward Program staff.
Client details	Not available
Sponsor/funding	National Guard

Table D.13
Operational Stress Injury Social Support

Feature	Description
Website/online documentation	http://www.vac-acc.gc.ca/general/sub.cfm?source=department/press/back_ground/osiss_program
Concept	A nonclinical approach to resilience and recovery from operational stress injuries (OSI), especially PTSD, depression, and anxiety disorders. Complementary to existing clinical treatments.
Mission	To establish, develop, and improve social support programs for members of the CF, veterans, and their families affected by operational stress. To provide education and training in the CF community to create an understanding and acceptance of operational stress injuries.
Background	Created in 2001 by Lieutenant-Colonel Stéphanie Grenier. Based on a peer support network of staff and volunteers originally set up by a small group of veterans. Extended to include military family members in 2005.
Resilience content	Social
Target audience	Military members and families (including bereaved families)
Phases of military deployment addressed	Post-deployment
Services	(1) OSISS members provide mirroring, empathy, and active listening for military members and their families. They also provide information about mental health resources. (2) OSISS members provide in-person support, such as accompanying service members to medical appointments.
Mode of delivery and dose	Individual and group support through face-to-face meetings and/or phone calls, typically every two weeks. Online resources are available.
Location of services	Canada
Staff	Currently, there are 40 to 45 OSISS staff members across Canada.
Training requirements of staff	Peer support coordinators require two weeks of training in total. Four days of this training are delivered by a psychologist through the Veterans Affairs Center. Peer support helpers require four days of training.
Client details	To date, OSISS has been provided to approximately 4,500 clients.
Sponsor/funding	Department of National Defense and Veterans Affairs Canada

Table D.14
Passport Toward Success

Feature	Description
Website/online documentation	http://apps.mhf.dod.mil/pls/psgprod/p?n=11087528715254401
Concept	A reunion support program with activities for learning and practicing skills to help children and families reconnect after a military deployment. Program addresses connection, communication, and stress during reintegration. Based on a social cognitive learning model and family systems theory.
Mission	To help children and families build skills to face the challenges of military deployment. To increase capacity of children and families to foster closer ties to family, friends, and the community. To promote strategies to attend to physical, mental, and emotional needs. To increase capacity to share and respond to feelings.
Background	This program was developed by the Military Family Research Institute (MFRI) at Purdue University in collaboration with the Indiana National Guard as part of the Yellow Ribbon Reintegration program.
Resilience content	Mental, social
Target audience	Children, adolescents, and families in the Indiana National Guard
Phases of military deployment addressed	Primarily post-deployment
Services	Children are divided into age groups and participate in activities with each other, then also with their parents. Groups rotate through "islands" with activities that focus on (1) feelings, (2) relaxation, and (3) communication.
Mode of delivery and dose	One-on-one meetings and support groups. The program is typically one day in duration but can be adapted to shorter versions.
Location of services	Throughout Indiana, the program is delivered in varied locations (e.g., hotel rooms, churches, tents, etc).
Staff	(1) Program coordinators are MFRI staff. (2) Program facilitators are bachelor- and masters-level social service providers who implement activities with children and families. (3) Program volunteers are nonmilitary community members and are screened by FBI checks, exams, and in-person training.
Training requirements of staff	Online training with five modules and a skills assessment. Additional on-site training is also available.
Client details	Children, adolescents, and families in the Indiana National Guard
Sponsor/funding	Purdue University and Indiana National Guard

Table D.15
The Penn Resiliency Project Master Resilience Training

Feature	Description
Website/online documentation	http://www.army.mil/csf/ http://www.ppc.sas.upenn.edu/prpsum.htm
Concept	Standardized resilience training that is based on cognitive-behavioral and positive psychology techniques. The program uses Ellis' Adversity-Consequences-Beliefs (ABC) model and has evolved based empirical research results.
Mission	PRP: To provide cognitive-behavioral and social problem-solving skills to improve individuals' ability to make decisions and cope with difficult situations. MRT: To complete a training support program and build a cadre of resiliency trainers for the force within five years. To increase overall resilience in the force by enhancing soldiers in the following dimensions: physical, social, spiritual, and family.
Background	PRP resilience programs were originally developed for middle school students and young adults. The first version of a manual for standardizing workshop delivery was published in 1991. Since 2007, a Train-the-Trainer model has enabled larger-scale dissemination of programs. PRP is currently one of three programs being integrated into the Army's CSF program.
Resilience content	Mental, social, spiritual
Target audience	Youth, young adults, students, executives, leaders, military service members, and their families
Phases of military deployment addressed	All phases
Services	(1) PRP: Workshop topics include recognizing and replacing automatic negative thoughts, behavioral activation strategies (e.g., graded task breakdown, antiprocrastination techniques), interpersonal skills (e.g., active listening, perspective-taking), stress management, generalizing coping skills to novel situations, developing character strengths, and positive communication. (2) MRT: Training specified for soldiers to increase core competencies in optimism, mental agility, self-regulation, self-awareness, self-efficacy, and connection. (3) Curriculum has also been developed specifically for youth (i.e., Positive Psychology for Youth Project).
Mode of delivery and dose	Face-to-face group workshops include rapport-building, didactic and multimedia presentations, participant role-playing, games and activities, group discussions, and homework reviews. MRT training is ten days in duration. Break-out sessions are led by one trainer and 4–5 facilitators. Leaders are then trained to teach learned skills to other soldiers.
Location of services	MRT training is currently available at the University of Pennsylvania and Ft. Jackson Victory University.
Staff	PRP co-director Reivich, facilitators, and trainers. For MRT, Reivich has trained approximately 40 facilitators (Army and civilian) and 15 trainers to date.

Table D.15—Continued

Feature	Description
Training requirements of staff	Leaders must learn the structured manual and receive 48 hours of training with Reivich. Reivich also supervises workshops to ensure adherence to the manual.
Client details	PRP has trained over 1,000 educators and clinicians in the U.S., UK, and Australia, including teachers and senior executives and manager from the Australian Federal Department of Education, Employment and Workplace Relations. Over 2,000 children and adolescents have attended PRP workshops. In August 2009, MRT was provided to 50 noncommissioned officers (NCOs). Since November 2009, 150–180 NCOs per month have been trained by the University of Pennsylvania, Ft. Jackson Victory University, and by teleconference.
Sponsor/funding	PRP: National Institute of Mental Health. MRT: Army.

Table D.16
Preventive Psychological Health Demonstration Project

Feature	Description
Website/online documentation	Not available
Concept	Program evaluations of three levels of resilience interventions for military populations (i.e., organizational, individual, and embedded/unit) to determine successful interventions for proactively preventing and treating psychological injury.
Mission	To extend service members' physical and mental endurance, to enhance physiological and psychological resilience, to reduce injury and illness, to mitigate risk for PTSD, to examine all factors that stress the deployed force, and to improve service members' success within the mental behavior domain.
Background	Program evaluations to be initiated by last quarter of FY 2009 and to continue until September 2011. Established in response to the Joint Force Health Protection Act of Concept of Operations (CONOPS) in July 2007.
Resilience content	Mental, physical
Target audience	Active-duty service members and family members
Phases of military deployment addressed	Predeployment, in theater, and post-deployment
Services	(1) Resilience Training Demonstration Project: To establish the effectiveness of psychological education interventions for service members. Biofeedback, stress reduction techniques, and mental skills training will be provided at the unit level, and outcome data will be compared with those from a matched cohort with no training. (2) Psychological Health Coordination Demonstration Project: To determine the efficacy of having an installation-level psychological health professional to coordinate the activities of mental health resources. Data collection is planned.
Mode of delivery and dose	Resilience training to be provided in person.
Location of services	Resilience training demonstration will occur at Ft. Hood, Tex. Psychological health coordination demonstration involves a senior commander and psychological health coordinator placed at Ft. Lewis, Ft. Hood, Ft. Bragg, Ft. Bliss, Ft. Drum, and Ft. Riley.
Staff	Council members for the demonstration projects include safety officers, chaplains, family advocacy staff, community service providers, sex assault advocates, safety officers, senior enlisted advisors, and mental health leaders.
Training requirements of staff	Coordinators require at least three weeks of training focused on organizational change.
Client details	Not applicable
Sponsor/funding	Department of Defense

Table D.17
Promoting Alternative THinking Strategies

Feature	Description
Website/online documentation	http://www.prevention.psu.edu/projects/PATHS.html
Concept	A research-based violence prevention program designed to facilitate the development of children's self-control, emotional awareness, and interpersonal problem-solving skills.
Mission	To help elementary-age children increase self-control, choose effective conflict-resolution strategies, reject aggressive responses to frustrating situations, and improve problem-solving skills.
Background	PATHS was founded in 1981 and initially provided services for children who are deaf. The program has been expanded to include children with and without special needs.
Resilience content	Mental, social
Target audience	Elementary-age children, their educators, and counselors
Phases of military deployment addressed	Not applicable
Services	Teachers, educators, and youth leaders deliver curricula to children with reference to six manuals that include over 100 interactive lessons. Lessons involve group discussions, role-playing skits, art activities, stories, and educational games. Topics addressed include self-control, feelings, relationships, and interpersonal cognitive problem-solving.
Mode of delivery and dose	Lessons are incorporated into existing in-person learning environments. Additional materials include "feelings" supplements, posters, and puppets. Lessons are generalized to everyday contexts in the classroom. Timing and frequency of sessions varies.
Location of services	International and U.S. classrooms (across approximately 25 states).
Staff	U.S. core staff comprises one full-time and 15 part-time employees. Core staff members train classroom teachers, other educators, and youth leaders to deliver this program to children.
Training requirements of staff	Core staff members require a minimum of three years of experience as PATHS teachers or consultants, participate in specialized training workshops, and receive certification after workshop observation.
Client details	International and U.S. schools and agencies, including military schools in Ft. Bragg and elsewhere
Sponsor/funding	Program is purchased by a school or community agency.

Table D.18
School Mental Health Team

Feature	Description
Website/online documentation	http://www.tamc.amedd.army.mil/offices/Psychiatry/smht.htm
Concept	A multidisciplinary team approach to promoting mental health within children's typical community of care. Providers (e.g., social workers, psychologists, and psychiatrists) work in coordination with school personnel.
Mission	To provide cost-effective, comprehensive, school-based mental health programs and services to support children, families, and military communities.
Background	Formerly called the Army School-Based Program, SMHT has been fully clinically operational since October 1998.
Resilience content	Mental, social
Target audience	Youth, parents, and staff at schools in military communities
Phases of military deployment addressed	Predeployment, in theater, and post-deployment
Services	(1) The School Wellness for Education Program is a Train-the-Trainer model for teachers, clients, and mental health professionals. (2) Clinical programs are available and provide adjunct services for students and families to address emotional and behavioral difficulties. (3) Training is available for students, families, and school staff to develop skills that promote positive functioning. (4) Deployment, parenting, and acculturation support and educational groups are also available.
Mode of delivery and dose	Services are provided face to face for individuals and groups. Some services are one time only, and others are ongoing (e.g., support groups).
Location of services	Three elementary schools and one middle school on Schofield Barracks, Oahu, Hawaii. Another elementary school on Marine Corps Base, Hawaii. (Expansion plans are currently underway.)
Staff	One psychologist as an administrator (assistant director), one child/adolescent psychiatrist, one clinical psychologist, and three clinical social workers. Second-year child/adolescent psychiatry fellows also provide limited supervised clinical duties.
Training requirements of staff	An intensive four-day program directed by the Military Child and Adolescent Center of Excellence was recently developed.
Client details	From July to September 2009, SMHT had active caseloads for approximately 128 children.
Sponsor/funding	Congress (through PTSD/TBI/BH funding)

Table D.19
Senior Leader Wellness Enhancement Seminar

Feature	Description
Website/online documentation	Not available
Concept	Senior leaders often take care of subordinates at the expense of themselves and their families. Seminars provide a proactive approach to help senior leaders and their spouses deal with their unique military-related challenges in a protected space.
Mission	To provide senior leaders and their spouses an opportunity to deal with their unique stressors and to "reset the force" from the top down. To destigmatize mental health illnesses starting with senior leaders and their spouses.
Background	Based on a seminar prepared for a single event. This program was cancelled in March 2008.
Resilience content	Social
Target audience	Senior military leaders and their spouses
Phases of military deployment addressed	Predeployment, in theater, and post-deployment
Services	The seminar content evolved over time. Topics included coping with leader stress, identifying and mitigating deployment-related stress, preamble to separation, reunion and reintegration, and dealing with combat grief and loss.
Mode of delivery and dose	Seminars included 80 to 120 participants and were approximately three hours, including breakout sessions. Resource lists and stress cards were also provided.
Location of services	Not available
Staff	The core facilitator group comprised 16 to 24 clinical social workers and psychologists.
Training requirements of staff	Clinical credentials
Client details	Not available
Sponsor/funding	Army

Brief Program Descriptions   151

Table D.20
Soldier Evaluation for Life Fitness

Feature	Description
Website/online documentation	Not available
Concept	Behavioral health is incorporated as a routine component of the health readiness process for all soldiers returning to their home stations after deployment.
Mission	For all soldiers to have face-to-face contact with both physical and mental health providers 90 to 180 days after deployment. To provide a comprehensive mental health assessment, ensure opportunities for soldiers to identify mental health concerns, establish familiarity with the mental health treatment process, and reduce treatment stigma.
Background	SELF evolved out of the Soldier Wellness Assessment Pilot Program (SWAP), which began as a pilot in 2005 at Madigan Army Medical Center at Ft. Lewis, Wash. SWAP evaluated soldiers both pre- and post-deployment. In May 2009, SELF was also introduced at Tripler Army Medical Center's health clinic at Schofield Barracks, Hawaii.
Resilience content	Mental, physical, spiritual
Target audience	Soldiers
Phases of military deployment addressed	Post-deployment
Services	(1) Soldiers watch a video in which a brigade commander and soldiers discuss their experiences and challenges adjusting to returning home after deployment. (2) Soldiers then complete an online adaptive screening instrument. An algorithm determines the interview focus area, duration, and clinician requirements (e.g., doctoral level providers are paired with highest risk soldiers). (3) The clinician then meets with the soldier and recommends follow-up resources.
Mode of delivery and dose	Video presentation, an online adaptive survey, and face-to-face interview with a provider. Interview duration is typically 15 to 60 minutes. Future appointments are scheduled as necessary.
Location of services	Ft. Lewis, Wash., and Schofield Barracks, Hawaii
Staff	One-third of staff members are doctoral-level behavioral health providers. The remaining two-thirds are master-level providers. (Behavioral health–trained primary care providers may be authorized to meet with soldiers who do not report mental health concerns.)
Training requirements of staff	Detailed training materials available including sample interview protocols, checklists, and military culture information. Length of training varies by individual provider from one day to one week.
Client details	Ft. Lewis is calibrated to serve 70 soldiers per day but can serve 100–120 under surge capacity. From 2005 to 2009, 41,000 soldiers completed post-deployment assessments, and 16,000 were referred to treatment beyond SELF.
Sponsor/funding	Army

Table D.21
Spiritual Warrior Training Program

Feature	Description
Website/online documentation	http://chfolsom.com/
Concept	Unit morale is related to individual spiritual well-being, which involves emotions, will, thoughts, faith, and purpose in life. Program principles are: (1) strength comes from hardship; (2) always give a way to escape; (3) faith-based (themes of reconciliation, forgiveness and purpose); (4) cohesion and morale; and (5) focus on serving others.
Mission	To apply innovative spiritual-wellness principles to enhance the Warrior Ethos, expedite increased morale, facilitate team integration and elevate performance. At the same time, to reduce training failures, sick calls, and disciplinary actions within the initial training environment. To provide consistent and intentional ministry within the unit by identifying the needs, providing innovative solutions, and executing the plan. This analytic approach takes a proactive stance in anticipating and identifying critical weaknesses within the human readiness factor of the unit.
Background	Founded in October 2007. Originally intended as a brigade-wide required project but has always been at the battalion level with support from the brigade chaplain.
Resilience content	Mental, spiritual
Target audience	Soldiers in basic combat training (BCT), especially those identified as high-risk.
Phases of military deployment addressed	Pre- and post-deployment
Services	(1) During BCT, data are collected on soldiers' in-training unit morale and cohesion. Staff team members identify and visit with high-risk individuals to develop and enhance coping and interpersonal skills. Devotionals are provided for non–high-risk soldiers. (2) For soldiers leaving the army, staff team members teach coping skills and assess military members' expectations about reintegration. (3) Chaplains participate at key unit events and provide continuous feedback to commanders.
Mode of delivery and dose	Face-to-face meetings with individuals and groups. Online resources are also available.
Location of services	Ft. Knox, where incoming and outgoing soldiers are processed.
Staff	Unit ministry team comprises one battalion chaplain and one assistant.
Training requirements of staff	Not applicable
Client details	Since the program's inception, approximately 9,000 soldiers have been served.
Sponsor/funding	Army

Table D.22
Warrior Resiliency Program

Feature	Description
Website/online documentation	Not available
Concept	A preventive approach intended to strengthen individual service members, their families, their units, and communities, enhancing their ability to cope with stress. Resilience promotion involves a continuum of care from nonclinical to clinical settings.
Mission	To build and restore resilience among soldiers and their families, to identify and overcome gaps in military behavioral health for building and restoring resilience, and to transform the legacy of pathology-based mental health services into a resilience-oriented behavioral health care system. To improve the quality of care rendered to soldiers and their families who are suffering from deployment-related problems and PTSD.
Background	Founded in February 2008 in response to a solicitation for Congressional supplemental funds. WRP will be part of the core budget through the PALM defense health program that flows to medical treatment facilities (e.g., Brook Army Medical Center) and is thus viable for a minimum of five years.
Resilience content	Mental, physical
Target audience	Military members and their families
Phases of military deployment addressed	In theater and post-deployment
Services	(1) Clinical Services Division: WRP is establishing a community resiliency initiative at Ft. Hood to determine how principles of population health can be applied to behavioral problems in the military. A PTSD partial hospitalization program is also in development. Services are provided to build and restore resilience in soldiers and their families. (2) Combat-related stress disorder training is provided to soldiers, their families, and medical personnel. A school-based initiative (SBI) at Ft. Houston promotes behavioral health in elementary-aged children in military families. (3) Clinical research includes survey research and program evaluation.
Mode of delivery and dose	Telephone service is provided to military members and their families for help with behavioral health problems. Training is also provided in person.
Location of services	Staff members are located at San Antonio Military Medical Center (SAMMC), Brooke Army Medical Center (BAMC), and Wilford Hall Medical Center (WHMC). The Community Resilience Initiative is in Ft. Hood, Tex.
Staff	Primarily Army staff, also Air Force. There are 45 to 50 personnel in total.
Training requirements of staff	Not available
Client details	Not available
Sponsor/funding	Army

Table D.23
Warrior Resilience and Thriving

Program	Warrior Resilience and Thriving (WRT)
Website/online documentation	http://www.dcoe.health.mil/DCoEV2/Content/navigation/documents/warrior%20resilience%20and%20thriving_%20maj%20jarrett.pdf
Concept	Based on Warrior Ethos principles (FM 6-22), Army Leadership, Seven Army Values, cognitive and rational emotive behavior therapy (REBT) self-counseling, posttraumatic growth, and positive psychology. Also draws from Japanese Bushido and other warrior cultures.
Mission	To enhance resilience, thriving, and posttraumatic growth recognition in warriors and combat teams while in theater and at home.
Background	WRT was developed during OIF in 2005. Originally a standardized class called Warrior Resilience Training, its name was changed to Warrior Resilience and Thriving to distinguish it from other programs. Variations of the program include: Warrior Resilience Training (2005–2006); Warrior Family Resilience and Thriving (WFRT, 2007–present); Elite Warrior Resilience and Thriving (2007); Warrior Resilience and Thriving-Provider (WRT-P, 2005–present); Warrior Resilience and Thriving Instructor Trainer (WRT-IT) Course (2009–present).
Resilience content	Mental, spiritual
Target audience	Military members and their families
Phases of military deployment addressed	Primarily in theater. Also pre- and post-deployment.
Services	(1) Standardized 90-minute mobile training classes focused on standardized combat and operational stress inoculation, resiliency, thriving, and posttraumatic growth. (2) Other WRT groups include WRT Medic Gross-Training (OIF, 2005–2006) and the WFRT counseling group.
Mode of delivery and dose	The WRT class is a one-time 90-minute interactive presentation with slides that is copresented by officer and enlisted prevention team members. Ongoing support groups are also available. These typically involve 4–8 sessions.
Location of services	Ft. Sill and in theater
Staff	Original staff: Major Jarrett and one sergeant. Staff size: three people or fewer (with occasional additional providers) until February 2009.
Training requirements of staff	Voluntary peer-unit counselors are required to attend a certification course that is eight sessions in duration.
Client details	As of September 2008, over 4,500 military members participated in WRT classes provided by the 98th Combat Stress Control Multi-National Division Baghdad Prevention team in OIF.
Sponsor/Funding	No formal funding

Bibliography

Adler, A.B., C.A. Castro, and D. McGurk, "Time-Driven Battlemind Psychological Debriefing: A Group-Level Early Intervention in Combat," *Military Medicine*, Vol. 174, No. 1, 2009a, pp. 21–28.

Adler, Amy B., Paul D. Bliese, Dennis McGurk, Charles W. Hoge, and Carl A. Castro, "Battlemind Debriefing and Battlemind Training as Early Interventions with Soldiers Returning from Iraq: Randomized by Platoon," *Journal of Consulting and Clinical Psychology*, Vol. 77, No. 5, 2009b, pp. 928–940.

Ano, G.G., and E.B. Vasconcelles, "Religious Coping and Psychological Adjustment to Stress: A Meta-Analysis," *Journal of Clinical Psychology*, Vol. 61, No. 4, 2005, pp. 461–480.

Bonanno, G.A., "Loss, Trauma, and Human Resilience—Have We Underestimated the Human Capacity to Thrive after Extremely Aversive Events?," *American Psychologist*, Vol. 59, No. 1, January 2004, pp. 20–28.

Bonanno, George A., and Anthony D. Mancini, "The Human Capacity to Thrive in the Face of Potential Trauma," *Pediatrics*, Vol. 121, 2008, pp. 369–375.

Bronfenbrenner, U., "Toward an Experimental Ecology of Human Development," *American Psychologist*, Vol. 32, No. 7, 1977, pp. 513–531.

Cicchetti, D., and M. Lynch, "Toward an Ecological/Transactional Model of Community Violence and Child Maltreatment: Consequences for Children's Development," *Children and Violence*, Vol. 56, 1993, p. 96.

Connor, Kathryn M., "Assessment of Resilience in the Aftermath of Trauma," *Journal of Clinical Psychiatry*, Vol. 67, No. 2, 2006, pp. 46–49.

Connor, K.M., and J.R. Davidson, "Development of a New Resilience Scale: The Connor-Davidson Resilience Scale (Cd-Risc)," *Depression and Anxiety*, Vol. 18, No. 2, 2003, p. 76.

CSF-Global Assessment Tool, Army Live blog. As of August 19, 2010: http://armylive.dodlive.mil/index.php/2009/12/csf-global-assessment-tool/

Defense Centers of Excellence for Psychological Health and Traumatic Brain Injury, "Building a Culture of Resilience." As of December 29, 2009: http://www.dcoe.health.mil/Content/navigation/images/resilience_continuum.jpg

Department of Defense Task Force on Mental Health, "An Achievable Vision: Report of the Department of Defense Task Force on Mental Health," 2007.

Fredrickson, Barbara L., Michele M. Tugade, Christian E. Waugh, and Gregory R. Larkin, "What Good Are Positive Emotions in Crises? A Prospective Study of Resilience and Emotions Following the Terrorist Attacks on the United States on September 11th, 2001," *Journal of Personality and Social Psychology*, Vol. 84, No. 2, 2003, pp. 365–376.

Friborg, O., O. Hjemdal, J.H. Rosenvinge, and M. Martinussen, "A New Rating Scale for Adult Resilience: What Are the Central Protective Resources Behind Healthy Adjustment?" *International Journal of Methods in Psychiatric Research*, Vol. 12, No. 2, 2003, pp. 65–76.

Garmezy, N., "Resiliency and Vulnerability to Adverse Developmental Outcomes Associated with Poverty," *American Behavioral Scientist*, Vol. 34, No. 4, 1991, pp. 416–430.

Helmus, T.C., and R.W. Glenn, *Steeling the Mind: Combat Stress Reactions and Their Implications for Urban Warfare*, Santa Monica, Calif.: RAND Corporation, MG-191-DA, 2005.

Jensen, Jeffrey M., and Mark W. Fraser, "A Risk and Resilience Framework for Child, Youth, and Family Policy," in *Social Policy for Children and Families: A Risk and Resilience Perspective*, Jensen, Jeffrey M., and Mark W. Fraser, eds., Thousand Oaks, Calif.: Sage Publications, 2005.

Jex, S.M., and P.D. Bliese, "Efficacy Beliefs as a Moderator of the Impact of Work-Related Stressors: A Multilevel Study," *Journal of Applied Psychology*, Vol. 84, No. 3, June 1999, pp. 349–361.

Judkins, S., et al., "Hardiness Training Among Nurse Managers: Building a Healthy Workplace," *Journal of Continuing Education in Nursing*, Vol. 37, 2006, pp. 202-207.

Kobasa, S.C., and S.R. Maddi, "Existential Personality Theory," in R.J. Corsini (Ed.), *Current Personality Theories*, Illinois: Peacock, 1977, pp. 243–276.

Lepore, Stephen, and Tracey Revenson, "Relationships Between Posttraumatic Growth and Resilience: Recovery, Resistance, and Reconfiguration" in *Handbook of Posttraumatic Growth: Research and Practice*, Calhoun, Lawrence G., and Richard G. Tedeschi, eds., Mahwah, NJ: Lawrence Erlbaum Associates, 2006.

Letourneau, Nicole, Jane Drummond, Darcy Fleming, Gerard Kysela, Linda McDonald, and Miriam Stewart, "Supporting Parents: Can Intervention Improve Parent-Child Relationships?," *Journal of Family Nursing*, Vol. 7, No. 2, May 1, 2001, pp. 159–187.

Lincoln, Y.S., and E.G. Guba, *Naturalistic Inquiry*, Thousand Oaks, Calif.: Sage Publications, 1985.

Loehr, J., and T. Schwartz, "The Making of a Corporate Athlete," *Harvard Business Review*, Vol. 79, No. 1, 2001, pp. 120–129.

Luthar, Suniya S., Dante Cicchetti, and Bronwyn Becker, "The Construct of Resilience: Implications for Interventions and Social Policies," *Child Development*, Vol. 71, No. 3, 2000, pp. 543–562.

Lynch, P.D., R. Eisenberger, and S. Armeli, "Perceived Organizational Support: Inferior Versus Superior Performance by Wary Employees," *Journal of Applied Psychology*, Vol. 84, 1999, pp. 467–483.

MacDermid, S.M., R. Samper, R. Schwarz, J. Nishida, and D. Nyaronga, *Understanding and Promoting Resilience in Military Families*, West Lafayette: Military Family Research Institute at Purdue University, 2008.

Maddi, S.R., et al., "Hardiness Training Facilitates Performance in College," *Journal of Positive Psychology*, Vol. 4, 2009, pp. 566–577.

Mancini, Anthony D., and George A. Bonanno, "Resilience in the Face of Potential Trauma: Clinical Practices and Illustrations," *Journal of Clinical Psychology*, Vol. 62, No. 8, 2006, pp. 971–985.

Martin Seligman's Positive Psychology Center, home page, 2007. As of September 26, 2010: http://www.ppc.sas.upenn.edu

Masten, A.S., "Resilience in Individual Development: Successful Adaptation Despite Risk and Adversity," *Educational Resilience in Inner-City America: Challenges and Prospects*, 1994, pp. 3–25.

Masten, A.S., K.M. Best, and N. Garmezy, "Resilience and Development: Contributions from the Study of Children Who Overcome Adversity," *Development and Psychopathology*, Vol. 2, No. 4, 1990, pp. 425–444.

Merriam-Webster Online, "Resilience," 2010. As of December 30, 2009:
http://www.merriam-webster.com/dictionary/RESILIENCE

National Association of Cognitive-Behavioral Therapists, home page, 2009. As of September 26, 2010:
http://www.nacbt.org

Norris, Fran H., Susan P. Stevens, Betty Pfefferbaum, Karen F. Wyche, and Rose L. Pfefferbaum, "Community Resilience as a Metaphor, Theory, Set of Capacities, and Strategy for Disaster Readiness," *American Journal of Community Psychology*, Vol. 41, 2008, pp. 127–150.

Nucifora, F., A.M. Langlieb, E. Siegal, G.S. Everly, and M. Kaminsky, *Building Resistance, Resilience, and Recovery in the Wake of School and Workplace Violence*: Department of Psychiatry and Behavioral Health Sciences, Johns Hopkins University School of Medicine, September 2007.

Punamaki, R.L., S. Qouta, E. El Sarraj, and E. Montgomery, "Psychological Distress and Resources Among Siblings and Parents Exposed to Traumatic Events," *International Journal of Behavioral Development*, Vol. 30, No. 5, September 2006, pp. 385–397.

Rachman, S.J., *Fear and Courage*. W.H. Freeman: San Francisco, 1978.

Rosenberg, M., "The Measurement of Self-Esteem," *Society and the Adolescent Self Image*, 1965, pp. 297–307.

Ryan, G.W., and H.R. Bernard, "Techniques to Identify Themes," *Field Methods*, Vol. 15, No. 1, 2003, p. 85.

Ryff, C.D., and C.L.M. Keyes, "The Structure of Psychological Well-Being Revisited," *Journal of Personality and Social Psychology*, Vol. 69, 1995, pp. 719–727.

Sammons, M.T., "Psychology in the Public Sector: Addressing the Psychological Effects of Combat in the US Navy," *American Psychologist*, Vol. 60, No. 8, 2005, pp. 899–909.

Schwartz, Tony, "Manage Your Energy, Not Your Time," *Harvard Business Review*, Vol. 85, No. 10, 2007, pp. 63–73.

Seligman, M.E., and M. Csikszentmihalyi, "Positive Psychology: An Introduction," *American Psychologist*, Vol. 55, No. 1, 2000, pp. 5–14.

Sinclair, V.G., and K.A. Wallston, "The Development and Psychometric Evaluation of the Brief Resilient Coping Scale," *Assessment*, Vol. 11, No. 1, 2004, p. 94.

Snyder, C.R., and S.J. Lopez, *Positive Psychology: The Scientific and Practical Explorations of Human Strengths*, Thousand Oaks, Calif.: Sage Publications, 2006.

Tanielian, Terri, and Lisa H. Jaycox, eds., *Invisible Wounds of War: Psychological and Cognitive Injuries, Their Consequences, and Services to Assist Recovery*, Santa Monica, Calif.: RAND Corporation, MG-720-CCF, 2008. As of April 30, 2010:
http://www.rand.org/pubs/monographs/MG720/

Tedeschi, R.G., and L.G. Calhoun, "Routes to Posttraumatic Growth Through Cognitive Processing," *Promoting Capabilities to Manage Posttraumatic Stress: Perspectives on Resilience*, 2003, pp. 12–26.

Tedeschi, Richard G., and Lawrence G. Calhoun, "Posttraumatic Growth: Conceptual Foundations and Empirical Evidence," *Psychological Inquiry*, Vol. 15, No. 1, 2004, pp. 1–15.

Wald, Jaye, Steven Taylor, Gordon J. Asmundson, Kerry L. Jang, and Jennifer Stapleton, *Literature Review of Concepts: Psychological Resiliency*, Vancouver, Canada: British Columbia University, 2006, http://handle.dtic.mil/100.2/ADA472961

Werner, E.E., "Resilience in Development," *Current Directions in Psychological Science*, 1995, pp. 81–85.

Wiens, Tina Watson, and Pauline Boss, "Maintaining Family Resiliency Before, During, and After Military Separation," in *Military Life: The Psychology of Serving in Peace and Combat*, Britt, Thomas W., Amy B. Adler, and Carl Andrew Castro, eds., Westport, Connecticut: Praeger Security International, 2006.

Zach, S., et al., "The Benefits of a Graduated Training Program for Security Officers on Physical Performance in Stressful Situations," *International Journal of Stress Management*, Vol. 14, 2007, pp. 350–369.